AAOS

Stephen J. Rahm, NREMT-P

EMT-Basic Review Manual
for National Certification

JONES AND BARTLETT PUBLISHERS

Sudbury, Massachusetts

BOSTON   TORONTO   LONDON   SINGAPORE

Jones and Bartlett Publishers

World Headquarters
Jones and Bartlett Publishers
40 Tall Pine Drive, Sudbury, MA 01776
978-443-5000
info@jbpub.com
www.EMSzone.com

Jones and Bartlett Publishers Canada
6339 Ormindale Way
Mississauga, ON CANADA L5V 1J2

Jones and Bartlett Publishers International
Barb House, Barb Mews
London W6 7PA, UK

Production Credits

Chief Executive Officer: Clayton E. Jones
Chief Operating Officer: Donald W. Jones, Jr.
President, Higher Education and Professional Publishing:
  Robert W. Holland, Jr.
V.P. Sales and Marketing: William J. Kane
V.P. Production and Design: Anne Spencer
V.P. Manufacturing and Inventory Control: Therese Connell
Publisher: Kimberly Brophy
Editor: Jennifer Reed
Production Editor: Karen Ferreira
Director of Marketing: Alisha Weisman
Text and Cover Design: Anne Spencer
Typesetting and Editorial: Carlisle Publishers Services
Printing and Binding: Courier Company

ISBN-13: 978-0-7637-4466-3
ISBN-10: 0-7637-4466-2

Library of Congress Cataloging in-Publication Data

Rahm, Stephen J.
  EMT-basic review manual for national certification / Stephen J. Rahm; American Academy of Orthopaedic Surgeons.
    p. ; cm.
  Includes bibliographical references and index.
  ISBN 0-7637-1829-7
  1. Emergency medicine—Examinations, questions, etc. 2. Emergency medicine—Outlines, syllabi, etc. I. Title
  [DNLM: 1. Emergency Medical Services—methods—Examination Questions. 2. Emergency Medical Technicians—standards—Examination Questions. 3. Emergency Treatment—methods—Examination Question. W 18.2 R147e2003]
  RC86.9.R345 2003
  616.02'076—dc21
  6048   2003040121
    Printed in the United States of America
    10 09   14 13 12 11

Contents

Acknowledgments

Jones and Bartlett Publishers and the author would like to thank the following individuals for their time, expertise, and assistance with this series.

Michael T. Czarnecki
Brooklyn, NY

Jonathan Epstein
Needham, MA

Diane Moore
Ft. Gordon, GA

Steve Carrier
White River Junction, VT

─────── **Dedication** ───────
For the honesty and integrity that they instilled in me throughout my
upbringing, this text is dedicated to my parents, Ann and Charles Rahm.
I will forever love them.

Stephen

Additional Credits

Unless otherwise indicated, photographs and illustrations have been supplied by the American Academy of Orthopaedic Surgeons, Jones and Bartlett Publishers, Stephen J. Rahm, and the Maryland Institute of Emergency Medical Services System.

Section Opener 2
© Richard Shock/Stone Images/Getty One

Section Opener 3, Skill Station 1
© Eddie Sperling

Preface

This review manual has been developed to prepare you for both the written and practical phases of the national EMT-Basic certification examination, which is based on the 1994 EMT-Basic National Standard Curriculum.

It is important to note that this manual is not an educational tool, but rather a review and assessment of your baseline knowledge. If used as intended, you will be able to identify any area(s) of weakness that you may have, thus allowing you to adjust your pre-examination studies accordingly.

No part of this review manual will guarantee success on any part of the national certification exam process. However, if used as an adjunct to regular study and practice, your chances of success are maximized.

Section 1 of this manual provides an overview of the 1994 EMT-Basic National Standard Curriculum (NSC).

Section 2 provides you with a series of practice written examinations that are designed to stimulate your critical thinking and problem solving skills, both of which are crucial attributes that EMS providers at all levels must possess.

Section 3 will review all of the skills that you are required to successfully complete as part of the national EMT-Basic examination process. For each skill, you will find helpful information, tips, and pointers designed to facilitate your progression through the practical examination.

Section 4 provides answers with detailed rationales for the practice written examinations.

All information contained within this review manual is based on the 1994 EMT-Basic National Standard Curriculum and the 2005 Emergency Cardiac Care (ECC) guidelines for basic cardiac life support.

For further information and resources, you can visit the following websites:

- Jones and Bartlett Publishers: www.EMSzone.com
- Emergency Care and Safety Institute: www.ECSinstitute.org
- National Registry of EMTs: www.nremt.org
- U.S. Dept. of Transportation: www.nhtsa.dot.gov

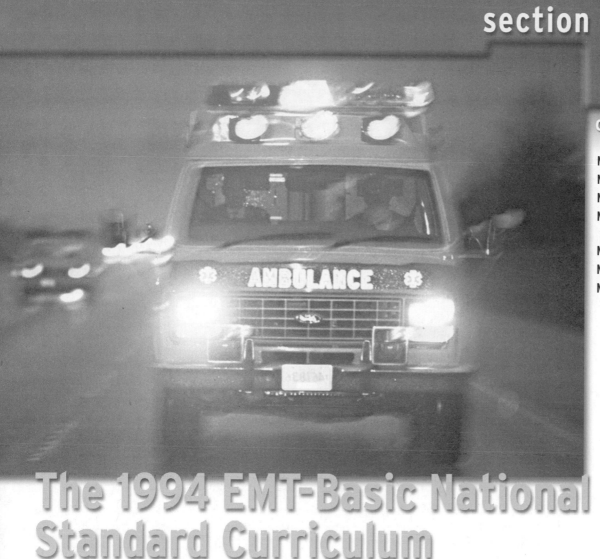

The 1994 EMT-Basic National Standard Curriculum

Each terminal objective of the 1994 EMT-Basic National Standard Curriculum (NSC) will be overviewed in this section.

The US DOT EMT-Basic National Standard Curriculum was last revised in 1994. The curriculum is a nationally recognized standard for providing basic level emergency medical care to the sick and injured patient. It is the foundation for prehospital emergency care from which you will build upon throughout your career in EMS. Though there are numerous textbooks that address prehospital care at the EMT-Basic level, they are all tools that allow you to achieve the standard as set forth by the US DOT. There are seven modules containing 32 lessons within the 1994 EMT-Basic National Standard Curriculum.

A well-rounded understanding of each of the curriculum modules and knowledge objectives will facilitate your overall understanding of your roles, responsibilities, and functions as an EMT-Basic. Furthermore, frequent practice of the psychomotor skills that are addressed later in this manual will prepare you to pass the EMT-Basic practical examination, which is designed to assess your ability to provide safe and effective emergency medical care to patients in the field.

Refer to your EMT-Basic textbook for the subobjectives for each module of the EMT-Basic curriculum. The entire 1994 EMT-Basic National Standard Curriculum can be downloaded from the National Highway Traffic Safety Administration (NHTSA) website at http://www.nhtsa.dot.gov

Module 1: Preparatory

Introduction to Emergency Medical Care

1-1 Familiarizes the EMT-Basic candidate with the introductory aspects of emergency medical care. Topics covered include the Emergency Medical Services (EMS) system, roles and responsibilities of the EMT-Basic, quality improvement, and medical direction.

Well-Being of the EMT-Basic

1-2 Covers the emotional aspects of emergency care, stress management, introduction to Critical Incident Stress Debriefing (CISD), scene safety, body substance isolation (BSI), personal protection equipment (PPE), and safety precautions that can be taken prior to performing the role of an EMT-Basic.

Medical/Legal and Ethical Issues

1-3 Explores the scope of practice, ethical responsibilities, advance directives, consent, refusals, abandonment, negligence, duty to act, confidentiality, and special situations such as organ donors and crime scenes. Medical/legal and ethical issues are vital elements of the EMT-Basic's daily life.

The Human Body

1-4 Enhances the EMT-Basic's knowledge of the human body. A brief overview of body systems, anatomy, physiology, and topographic anatomy will be given in this session.

Baseline Vital Signs and SAMPLE history.

1-5 Teaches assessing and recording of a patient's vital signs and a SAMPLE history.

Lifting and moving patients

1-6 Provides students with knowledge of body mechanics, lifting and carrying techniques, principles of moving patients, and an overview of equipment. Practical skills of lifting and moving will also be developed during this lesson.

Module 2: Airway

Airway

2-1 Teaches airway anatomy and physiology, how to maintain an open airway, pulmonary resuscitation, and variations for infants and children and patients with laryngectomies. The use of airways, suction equipment, oxygen equipment and delivery systems, and resuscitation devices will be discussed in this lesson.

Module 3: Patient Assessment

Scene Size-Up

3-1 Enhances the EMT-Basic's ability to evaluate a scene for potential hazards, determine by the number of patients if additional help is necessary, and evaluate mechanism of injury or nature of illness. This lesson draws on the knowledge of Lesson 1-2.

Initial Assessment

3-2 Provides the knowledge and skills to properly perform the initial assessment. In this session, the student will learn about forming a general impression, determining responsiveness, assessment of the airway, and breathing and circulation. Students will also discuss how to determine priorities of patient care.

Baseline Vital Signs and SAMPLE History

3-3 Teaches assessment and recording of a patient's vital signs and SAMPLE history.

Focused History and Physical Exam–Trauma Patients

3-4 Describes and demonstrates the method of assessing patients' traumatic injuries. A rapid approach to the trauma patient will be the focus of this lesson.

Detailed Physical Exam

3-5 Teaches the knowledge and skills required to continue the assessment and treatment of the patient.

On-Going Assessment

3-6 Stresses the importance of trending, recording changes in the patient's condition, and reassessment of interventions to ensure appropriate care.

Communications

3-7 Discusses the components of a communication system, radio communications, communication with medical direction, verbal communication, interpersonal communication, and quality improvement.

Documentation

3-8 Assists the EMT-Basic in understanding the components of the written report, special considerations regarding patient refusal, the legal implications of the report, and special reporting situations. Reports are an important aspect of prehospital care. This skill will be integrated into all student practices.

Module 4: Medical Emergencies

General Pharmacology

4-1 Provides the student with a basic knowledge of pharmacology, providing a foundation for the administration of medications given by the EMT-Basic and those used to assist a patient with self-administration.

Respiratory Emergencies

4-2 Reviews components of the lesson on respiratory anatomy and physiology. It also will provide instruction on assessment of respiratory difficulty and emergency medical care of respiratory problems, and the administration of prescribed inhalers.

Cardiovascular Emergencies

4-3 Reviews of the cardiovascular system, an introduction to the signs and symptoms of cardiovascular disease, administration of a patient's prescribed nitroglycerin, and use of the automated external defibrillator.

Diabetes/Altered Mental Status

4-4 Reviews of the signs and symptoms of altered level of consciousness, the emergency medical care of a patient with signs and symptoms of altered mental status and a history of diabetes, and the administration of oral glucose.

Allergies

4-5 Teaches the student to recognize the signs and symptoms of an allergic reaction, and to assist the patient with a prescribed epinephrine auto-injector.

Poisoning/Overdose

4-6 Teaches the student to recognize the signs and symptoms of poisoning and overdose. Information on the administration of activated charcoal is also included in this section.

Environmental Emergencies

4-7 Teaches the student to recognize the signs and symptoms of heat and cold exposure, as well as the emergency medical care of these conditions. Information on aquatic emergencies and bites and stings also will be included in this lesson.

Behavioral Emergencies

4-8 Develops the student's awareness of behavioral emergencies and the management of the disturbed patient. Restraining the combative patient also will be taught in this lesson.

Obstetrics/Gynecology

4-9 Reviews the anatomical and physiological changes that occur during pregnancy, demonstrates normal and abnormal deliveries, summarizes signs and symptoms of common gynecological emergencies, and describes neonatal resuscitation.

Module 5: Trauma

Bleeding and Shock

5-1 Reviews the cardiovascular system, describes the care of the patient with internal and external bleeding, signs and symptoms of shock (hypoperfusion), and the emergency medical care of shock (hypoperfusion).

Soft-Tissue Injuries

5-2 Continues with the information taught in Lesson 5-1, Bleeding and Shock, discussing the anatomy of the skin and the management of soft-tissue injuries and the management of burns. Techniques of dressing and bandaging wounds also will be taught in this lesson.

Musculoskeletal Care

5-3 Includes reviews of the musculoskeletal system. Recognition of signs and symptoms of a painful, swollen, deformed extremity and splinting are taught in this section.

Injuries to the Head and Spine

5-4 Reviews the anatomy of the nervous and skeletal systems. Injuries to the spine and head, including mechanism of injury, signs and symptoms of injury, and assessment are discussed. Emergency medical care, including the use of cervical immobilization devices and short and long backboards also will be discussed and demonstrated by the instructor and students. Other topics include helmet removal and infant and child considerations.

Module 6: Infants and Children

Infants and Children

6-1 Presents information concerning the developmental and anatomical differences in infants and children, discusses common medical and trauma situations, and covers infants and children who are dependent on special technology. The challenge for EMS providers of dealing with an ill or injured infant or child patient also is discussed.

Module 7: Operations

Ambulance Operations

7-1 Presents an overview of the knowledge needed to function in the prehospital environment. Topics covered include responding to a call, emergency vehicle operations, transferring patients, and the phases of an ambulance call.

Gaining Access

7-2 Provides the EMT-Basic student with an overview of rescue operations. Topics covered include roles and responsibilities at a crash scene, equipment, gaining access, and removing the patient.

Overviews/Special Operations

7-3 Provides the EMT-Basic student with information about hazardous materials, incident management systems, mass-casualty situations, and basic triage.

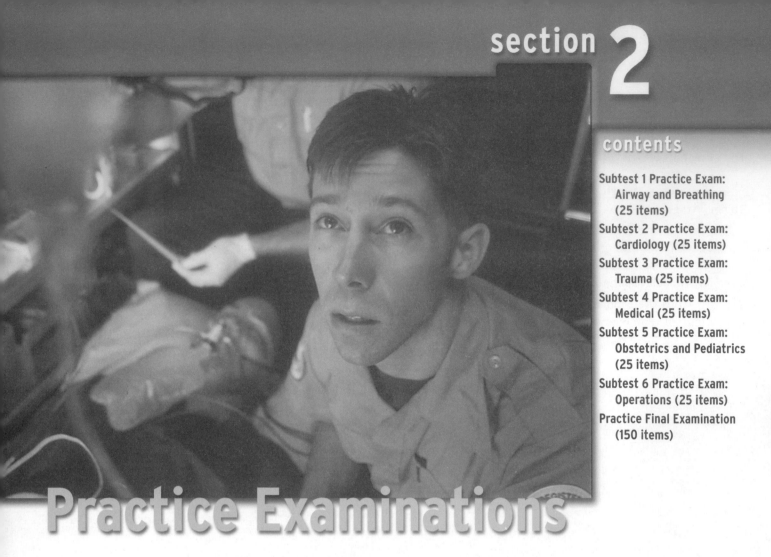

Practice Examinations

This section contains seven practice exams totaling 300 questions. The first six exams contain 25 questions each and represent the individual subtests that comprise the national EMT-Basic written examination. You should focus your preparatory studies in any area(s) that you answered seven or more questions incorrectly.

Following the individual subtests, you will take a comprehensive 150-item final practice exam, which reflects all six subtests in a scrambled fashion. At the end of the final practice exam, you will find a blueprint that categorizes each question into a subtest area and suggests a minimum number of correctly answered questions.

In order to obtain a reliable assessment of your baseline knowledge, it is highly recommended that you complete each individual test in its entirety prior to reading the correct answers and detailed rationales, which can be found in Section IV of this manual.

All practice questions in this section are based upon the following:
- 1994 US DOT EMT-Basic National Standard Curriculum.
- 2005 Emergency Cardiac Care (ECC) guidelines for basic cardiac life support.

Subtest I Practice Exam: Airway and Breathing

1. Which of the following statements regarding the head tilt-chin lift maneuver is most correct?
   a. It can only be used in conjunction with an oropharyngeal airway.
   b. It can only be used temporarily and must be replaced by an airway adjunct.
   c. It should be used on all unresponsive patients that you encounter.
   d. It is the technique of choice for patients with potential spinal injury.

2. In which of the following situations should the jaw-thrust maneuver be used?
   a. In any patient who is in cardiac arrest
   b. In a patient with apnea with no signs of trauma
   c. In a patient who is in need of frequent suctioning
   d. When the mechanism of injury is unclear

3. An elderly man is found lying unresponsive next to his bed. The patient's wife did not witness the event that caused the unconsciousness. You should first
   a. assess the patient's respirations.
   b. apply 100% supplemental oxygen.
   c. tilt the head back and lift up the chin.
   d. grasp the angles of the lower jaw and lift.

4. A patient has severe facial injuries, inadequate breathing, and copious secretions coming from the mouth. How should this situation be managed?
   a. Alternate suctioning for 15 seconds and ventilations for 2 minutes.
   b. Provide artificial ventilations and suction for 30 seconds as needed.
   c. Turn the patient to the side and provide oral suctioning continuously.
   d. Insert an oropharyngeal airway and suction until the secretions clear.

5. When ventilating an apneic adult patient with a bag-valve mask device, you must make sure that
   a. an airway adjunct has been inserted.
   b. you are positioned alongside the patient.
   c. ventilations occur at a rate of 20 breaths/min.
   d. the pop-off valve on the BVM device remains open.

6. Which of the following processes occurs during inhalation?
   a. The intercostal muscles and diaphragm both contract.
   b. The intercostal muscles relax and the diaphragm descends.
   c. The diaphragm contracts and the intercostal muscles relax.
   d. The diaphragm descends and the intercostal muscles relax.

7. Which of the following processes occurs during cellular/capillary gas exchange?
   a. The cells give up oxygen to the capillaries.
   b. The cells receive carbon dioxide from the capillaries.
   c. The capillaries give up oxygen to the cells.
   d. The capillaries give up carbon dioxide to the cells.

_____ **8.** What is the preferred method for initially providing artificial ventilations to a patient with apnea?
  a. Flow-restricted, oxygen-powered ventilation device
  b. Mouth-to-mask technique with supplemental oxygen
  c. One-person bag-valve-mask technique with 100% oxygen
  d. Two-person bag-valve-mask technique with 100% oxygen

_____ **9.** A reduced tidal volume would most likely occur from
  a. flaring of the nostrils.
  b. accessory muscle use.
  c. unequal chest expansion.
  d. increased minute volume.

_____ **10.** Which of the following patients is exhibiting signs of inadequate breathing?
  a. A 41-year-old woman with shallow respirations of 20 breaths/min
  b. A 60-year-old woman with bilaterally equal breath sounds
  c. A 30-year-old man with respirations of 18 breaths/min and equal breath sounds
  d. A 50-year-old man with respirations of 12 breaths/min and pink, dry skin

_____ **11.** Snoring respirations in an unresponsive patient most likely are the result of
  a. foreign body airway obstruction.
  b. upper airway obstruction by the tongue.
  c. collapse of the trachea during breathing.
  d. swelling of the larynx and surrounding structures.

_____ **12.** In an unresponsive patient who has not sustained trauma, how are respirations of 16 breaths/min with good chest expansion most appropriately managed?
  a. Suctioning as needed and artificial ventilations
  b. The jaw-thrust maneuver and frequent suctioning
  c. An airway adjunct and oxygen via nonrebreathing mask
  d. An airway adjunct and ventilations with a BVM device

_____ **13.** Initial management of an unconscious adult patient who fell 15′ from a tree includes
  a. performing a jaw-thrust maneuver.
  b. performing a head tilt-chin lift maneuver.
  c. providing oxygen or artificial ventilations.
  d. assessing the rate and quality of breathing.

_____ **14.** What should your first action be when treating a 40-year-old man with rapid respirations?
  a. Apply 100% supplemental oxygen.
  b. Insert an airway adjunct as needed.
  c. Assess the regularity and quality of breathing.
  d. Initiate artificial ventilations with a pocket mask.

_____ **15.** In what position would you expect a patient with severe dyspnea to be in?
  a. Prone
  b. Supine
  c. Fowler's
  d. Lateral recumbent

16. Which of the following listings of techniques and devices represents the correct order of preference for providing artificial ventilation?
   a. Pocket mask, one-person BVM, two-person BVM, flow-restricted oxygen-powered ventilation device
   b. Pocket mask, two-person BVM, flow-restricted oxygen-powered ventilation device, one-person BVM
   c. One-person BVM, pocket mask, two-person BVM, flow-restricted oxygen-powered ventilation device
   d. Two-person BVM, one-person BVM, flow-restricted oxygen-powered ventilation device, pocket mask

17. Tidal volume is best defined as the
   a. volume of air inhaled in a single breath.
   b. volume of air that remains in the upper airway.
   c. total volume of air that the lungs are capable of holding.
   d. volume of air moved in and out of the lungs each minute.

18. You would most likely encounter agonal respirations in which of the following patients?
   a. A hypoxic patient who is in the early phase of compensation
   b. A severely hypoxic patient who is in the later stages of compensation
   c. A patient who is in the midst of complete respiratory failure
   d. A semiconscious patient whose tongue is occluding the airway

19. A young woman who has overdosed on a strong narcotic drug is unconscious with slow, shallow breathing. As you attempt to insert an oropharyngeal airway, the patient begins to gag. You should next
   a. remove the oropharyngeal airway and be prepared to suction the mouth.
   b. remove the oropharyngeal airway and insert a nasopharyngeal airway.
   c. suction the patient's oropharynx as you insert a nasopharyngeal airway.
   d. make sure you are using the most appropriate size of oropharyngeal airway.

20. As you are ventilating an apneic patient using the one-person bag-valve-mask technique, you note minimal rise of the chest each time you squeeze the bag. You should
   a. ensure that the reservoir is attached to the bag-valve-mask device.
   b. squeeze the bag harder to ensure delivery of adequate tidal volume.
   c. suction the patient's mouth for 15 seconds and reattempt ventilations.
   d. evaluate the mask-to-face seal and the position of the patient's head.

21. After an adult cardiac arrest patient has been intubated by a paramedic, you are providing ventilations as your partner performs chest compressions. When ventilating the patient, you should
   a. deliver 2 breaths during a brief pause in chest compressions.
   b. deliver each breath over 1 second at a rate of 8 to 10 breaths/min.
   c. hyperventilate the patient to maximize carbon dioxide elimination.
   d. deliver each breath over 2 seconds at a rate of 12 to 15 breaths/min.

_____ 22. When ventilating a patient with apnea with a pocket mask device, each breath should be delivered over
   a. 1 second.
   b. 2 seconds.
   c. 3 seconds.
   d. 4 seconds.

_____ 23. A 60-year-old woman presents with acute respiratory distress. She is alert and oriented, but restless. Her respiratory rate is 26 breaths/min with adequate chest expansion and clear breath sounds. What is the most appropriate method of airway management for this patient?
   a. Supplemental oxygen with a nonrebreathing mask
   b. A nasopharyngeal airway and assisted ventilations
   c. A nasopharyngeal airway and supplemental oxygen
   d. A nasal cannula with the flowmeter set at 4 to 6 L/min

_____ 24. A semiconscious young man has shallow, gurgling respirations at a rate of 10 breaths/min. Initial management should include
   a. suctioning the oropharynx.
   b. inserting a nasopharyngeal airway.
   c. initiating positive pressure ventilations.
   d. applying 100% oxygen with a nonrebreathing mask.

_____ 25. Which of the following airway sounds would most likely indicate a lower airway obstruction?
   a. Stridor
   b. Crowing
   c. Gurgling
   d. Wheezing

Subtest 2 Practice Exam: Cardiology

23/25 Q21.

_____ 1. Which of the following assessment findings would most likely indicate cardiac compromise?
   a. Tachypnea
   b. Tachycardia
   c. Irregular pulse
   d. Sudden fainting

_____ 2. A 50-year-old man presents with "crushing" chest pain of sudden onset. He is diaphoretic and nauseated. You should
   a. obtain baseline vital signs.
   b. apply supplemental oxygen.
   c. ask him if he takes nitroglycerin.
   d. perform a focused physical exam.

B ✓

3. As you are assessing an elderly man who is complaining of chest pain, the patient suddenly loses consciousness. Your first step should be to
  a. attach the AED.
  b. open the airway.
  c. assess for a pulse.
  d. assess for breathing.

C ✓

4. Freshly oxygenated blood returns to the heart via which of the following blood vessels?
  a. Aorta
  b. Vena cava
  c. Pulmonary vein
  d. Pulmonary artery

D ✓

5. Which of the following statements regarding the automated external defibrillator is true?
  a. It should be applied to patients at risk for cardiac arrest
  b. It will analyze a patient's rhythm while CPR is in progress
  c. It should not be used in patients with an implanted pacemaker
  d. It can safely be used in children between 1 and 8 years of age

A ✓

6. Nitroglycerin possesses which of the following effects when administered to patients with suspected cardiac chest pain?
  a. Vasodilation and increased myocardial oxygen supply
  b. Vasodilation and decreased myocardial oxygen supply
  c. Vasoconstriction and increased cardiac workload
  d. Vasoconstriction and increased cardiac oxygen demand

————— **Questions 7 to 9 apply to the following scenario:** —————

You arrive at the scene of a 56-year-old man who is not breathing. Your initial assessment reveals that the patient is pulseless and apneic. The patient's wife tells you that her husband suddenly grabbed his chest and then passed out.

C ✓

7. As your partner confirms cardiac arrest and begins one-rescuer CPR, you should
  a. notify medical control.
  b. insert an airway adjunct.
  c. prepare the AED for use.
  d. obtain a SAMPLE history. ✓

C

8. When performing two-rescuer CPR on this patient, you should
  a. slowly compress the chest to a depth of about 1" to 1 ½".
  b. not attempt to synchronize compressions with ventilations.
  c. have your partner pause after 30 compressions as you give two breaths.
  d. continue ventilations as the AED analyzes the patient's cardiac rhythm.

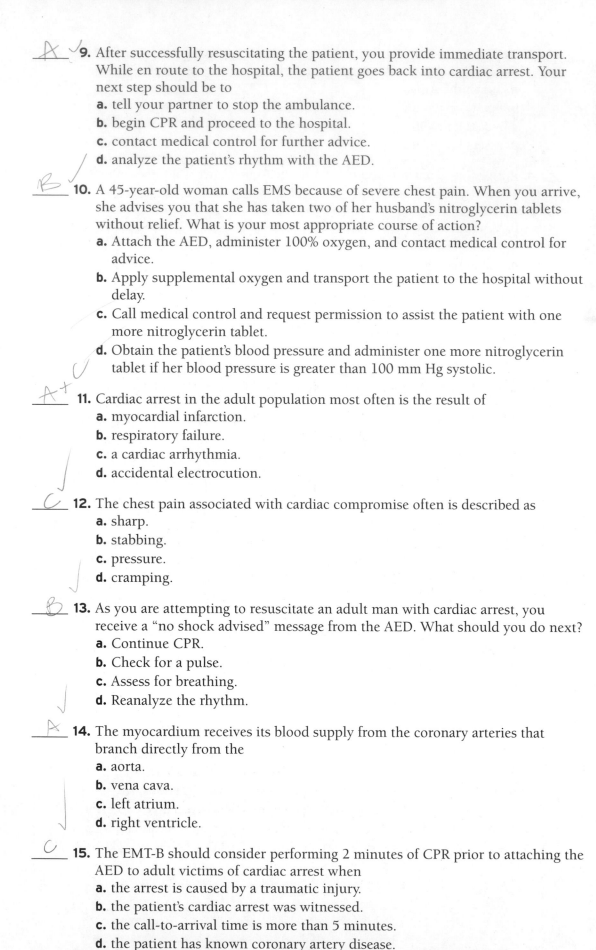

A   **9.** After successfully resuscitating the patient, you provide immediate transport. While en route to the hospital, the patient goes back into cardiac arrest. Your next step should be to
  a. tell your partner to stop the ambulance.
  b. begin CPR and proceed to the hospital.
  c. contact medical control for further advice.
  d. analyze the patient's rhythm with the AED.

B   **10.** A 45-year-old woman calls EMS because of severe chest pain. When you arrive, she advises you that she has taken two of her husband's nitroglycerin tablets without relief. What is your most appropriate course of action?
  a. Attach the AED, administer 100% oxygen, and contact medical control for advice.
  b. Apply supplemental oxygen and transport the patient to the hospital without delay.
  c. Call medical control and request permission to assist the patient with one more nitroglycerin tablet.
  d. Obtain the patient's blood pressure and administer one more nitroglycerin tablet if her blood pressure is greater than 100 mm Hg systolic.

A+   **11.** Cardiac arrest in the adult population most often is the result of
  a. myocardial infarction.
  b. respiratory failure.
  c. a cardiac arrhythmia.
  d. accidental electrocution.

C   **12.** The chest pain associated with cardiac compromise often is described as
  a. sharp.
  b. stabbing.
  c. pressure.
  d. cramping.

B   **13.** As you are attempting to resuscitate an adult man with cardiac arrest, you receive a "no shock advised" message from the AED. What should you do next?
  a. Continue CPR.
  b. Check for a pulse.
  c. Assess for breathing.
  d. Reanalyze the rhythm.

A   **14.** The myocardium receives its blood supply from the coronary arteries that branch directly from the
  a. aorta.
  b. vena cava.
  c. left atrium.
  d. right ventricle.

C   **15.** The EMT-B should consider performing 2 minutes of CPR prior to attaching the AED to adult victims of cardiac arrest when
  a. the arrest is caused by a traumatic injury.
  b. the patient's cardiac arrest was witnessed.
  c. the call-to-arrival time is more than 5 minutes.
  d. the patient has known coronary artery disease.

C **16.** Which of the following are side effects of nitroglycerin?
   a. Nausea
   b. Anxiety
   c. Headache
   d. Hypertension

B **17.** Which of the following patients would be the best candidate for the administration of nitroglycerin?
   a. A woman who has taken three doses of prescribed nitroglycerin without relief of chest pain
   b. A woman with chest pain, prescribed nitroglycerin, and a blood pressure of 102/76 mm Hg
   c. A man with chest pain, a bottle of expired nitroglycerin, and a blood pressure of 110/80 mm Hg
   d. An elderly man with crushing chest pain and a blood pressure of 90/60 mm Hg

C **18.** Which of the following chambers of the heart has the thickest walls?
   a. Left atrium
   b. Right atrium
   c. Left ventricle
   d. Right ventricle

B **19.** In addition to oxygen therapy, the most effective way to minimize the detrimental effects associated with cardiac compromise is to
   a. give the patient up to four doses of nitroglycerin.
   b. reassure the patient and provide prompt transport.
   c. transport the patient rapidly, using lights and siren.
   d. request ALS support for all patients who have chest pain.

A **20.** Which of the following questions would be most appropriate to ask when assessing a patient with chest pain?
   a. What does the pain feel like?
   b. Does the pain radiate to your arm?
   c. Would you describe the pain as sharp?
   d. Is the pain worse when you take a deep breath?

D **21.** Which of the following statements regarding one-rescuer CPR is correct?
   a. You should assess the patient for a pulse after 3 cycles of CPR.
   b. A compression to ventilation ratio of 15:2 should be delivered.
   c. Ventilations should be delivered over a period of 1 to 2 seconds.
   d. The chest should be allowed to fully recoil after each compression.

D **22.** You are caring for a 66-year-old woman with severe pressure in her chest. As you initiate oxygen therapy, your partner should
   a. notify medical control.
   b. obtain a SAMPLE history.
   c. measure the blood pressure.
   d. gather the patient's medications.

_B_ **23.** When managing a patient with chest pain, you should first
  a. administer high-concentration oxygen.
  b. place the patient in a position of comfort.
  c. request an ALS ambulance to respond to the scene.
  d. measure the blood pressure and administer nitroglycerin.

_B_ **24.** What is the most detrimental effect that tachycardia can have on a patient experiencing cardiac compromise?
  a. Increased blood pressure
  b. Increased oxygen demand
  c. Increased stress and anxiety
  d. Decreased cardiac functioning

_____ **25.** After applying the AED to a 56-year-old female in cardiac arrest, you analyze her cardiac rhythm and receive a "shock advised" message. First responders, who arrived at the scene before you, tell you that the patient was without CPR for about 10 minutes. You should
  a. perform 2 minutes of CPR and then defibrillate.
  b. detach the AED and prepare for immediate transport.
  c. deliver the shock as indicated followed immediately by CPR.
  d. notify medical control and request permission to cease resuscitation.

Subtest 3 Practice Exam: Trauma

_C_ **1.** During transport of a patient with a head injury, what assessment factor will provide you with the most information regarding the patient's condition?
  a. Pupil size
  b. Heart rate
  c. Mental status
  d. Blood pressure

_A_ **2.** A young man fell and landed on his outstretched hand, resulting in pain and deformity to the left midshaft forearm. Distal circulation should be assessed at which of the following pulse locations?
  a. Radial
  b. Brachial
  c. Pedal
  d. Popliteal

_A_ **3.** You are called to a local nightclub for an injured patient. Upon arrival, you see a young man who is lying on the ground screaming in pain; bright red blood is spurting from an apparent stab wound to his groin area. Your first action should be to
  a. control the bleeding.
  b. apply 100% oxygen.
  c. ensure an open airway.
  d. elevate the patient's legs.

4. During a soccer game, a 20-year-old man collided shoulder-to-shoulder with another player. He has pain and a noticeable anterior bulge to the left shoulder. What is the most effective method of immobilizing this injury?
  a. An air-inflatable splint with the left arm immobilized in the flexed position
  b. A long board splint with the left arm immobilized in the extended position
  c. A sling to support the left arm and swathes to secure the arm to the body
  d. A sling to support the left arm and swathes to maintain downward traction

5. Which of the following mechanisms of injury would necessitate performing a rapid trauma assessment?
  a. A 5'8" tall adult who fell 12' from a roof and landed on his side
  b. A stable patient involved in a car crash, whose passenger was killed
  c. Amputation of three toes from the patient's left foot with controlled bleeding
  d. An impaled object in the patient's lower extremity with minimal venous bleeding

6. You are assessing a 33-year-old male's Glasgow Coma Scale (GCS) score. The patient opens his eyes in response to pain, is speaking with incomprehensible words, and withdraws from pain by flexing his upper extremities. What is his GCS score?
  a. 6
  b. 7
  c. 8
  d. 9

──────── **Questions 7 to 9 pertain to the following scenario:** ────────
The police summon you to a residence for a domestic dispute. When you arrive, you are advised by a police officer that a man, who is now in custody, shot his wife. When you enter the residence, you see a woman lying supine. She is conscious, but very restless, and is in obvious respiratory distress.
───

7. After ensuring a patent airway, your next course of action should be to
  a. apply 100% oxygen.
  b. assess respiratory quality.
  c. compare carotid and radial pulses.
  d. check the condition of the patient's skin.

8. During which part of your assessment would you be most likely to discover a small caliber gunshot wound, with minimal bleeding, to the back?
  a. General impression
  b. Initial assessment
  c. Rapid trauma assessment
  d. Detailed physical examination

9. Upon discovering an open chest wound, your first action should be to
  a. prevent air from entering the open wound.
  b. begin assisted ventilation and prepare for transport.
  c. immediately reassess the patient's ventilatory status.
  d. cover the wound with a trauma dressing and reassess the patient's ventilatory status.

10. When applying a vest-style spinal immobilization device to a patient with traumatic neck pain, you should
  a. immobilize the head prior to securing the torso straps.
  b. secure the torso section prior to immobilizing the head.
  c. ask the patient to fully exhale as you secure the torso.
  d. gently flex the head forward as you position the device.

11. Which of the following findings would indicate that a patient is in decompensated shock?
  a. Diaphoresis and pallor
  b. Falling blood pressure
  c. Restlessness and anxiety
  d. Heart rate greater than 130 beats/min

12. General care for an amputated body part includes
  a. immersing the amputated part in cold water to prevent further damage.
  b. thoroughly cleaning the amputated part and wrapping it in a sterile dressing.
  c. wrapping the amputated part in a moist, sterile dressing and placing it on ice.
  d. wrapping the amputated part in a moist, sterile dressing and keeping it warm.

13. You are called to a local knife-throwing contest, where a 42-year-old man has a large dagger impaled in the middle of his chest. Your assessment reveals that he is pulseless and apneic. How should you manage this patient and his injury?
  a. Carefully remove the knife, control the bleeding, and begin CPR.
  b. Carefully remove the knife, control the bleeding, and attach an AED to the patient.
  c. Secure the knife in place with a bulky dressing and transport immediately.
  d. Make sure that the knife is secured, initiate CPR, and transport immediately.

14. Rapid extrication of a patient from an automobile is most appropriately performed by
  a. applying an extrication collar and removing the patient from the car using the direct carry method.
  b. applying an extrication collar, sliding a long spine board under the patient's buttocks, and removing the patient from the car.
  c. applying a vest-style extrication device and sliding the patient out of the car onto a long spine board for full immobilization.
  d. maintaining support of the head, grasping the patient by the clothing, and rapidly removing the patient from the car.

15. During your rapid trauma assessment of a critically-injured patient, you should assess the chest for
  a. symmetry and pain.
  b. rigidity and guarding.
  c. crepitus and distention.
  d. distention and guarding.

16. Following penetrating trauma to the abdomen, a 50-year-old woman has a large laceration with a loop of protruding bowel. How should you manage this injury?

   a. Carefully replace the bowel and apply an occlusive dressing.

   b. Carefully replace the bowel and cover the wound with a moist, sterile dressing.

   c. Apply a dry, sterile dressing covered by an occlusive dressing.

   d. Apply a moist, sterile dressing, covered by a dry, sterile dressing.

17. During the initial assessment of an unconscious trauma patient, you find that the patient is breathing inadequately, has a weak radial pulse, and is bleeding from a lower extremity wound. You should direct your partner to

   a. radio for an ALS ambulance to respond to the scene.

   b. apply direct pressure to the bleeding as you assist ventilations.

   c. initiate positive pressure ventilations as you control the bleeding.

   d. prepare the long spine board and straps for rapid immobilization.

18. While removing a hot radiator cap, a young man sustained partial-thickness burns to the anterior chest and both anterior arms. Based on the Rule of Nines, what percentage of his body surface area (BSA) has been burned?

   a. 18%

   b. 27%

   c. 36%

   d. 45%

19. An elderly woman who was removed from her burning house by firefighters has sustained full-thickness burns to approximately 50% of her body. Appropriate management for this patient should consist of

   a. applying moist, sterile dressings to the burned areas and preventing hypothermia.

   b. cooling the burns with sterile saline and covering them with dry, sterile burn pads.

   c. covering the burns with dry, sterile dressings and preventing further loss of body heat.

   d. peeling burned clothing from the skin and removing all rings, necklaces, and bracelets.

20. Initial care of a large avulsion includes

   a. cleaning the wound.

   b. controlling any bleeding.

   c. assessing distal circulation.

   d. immobilizing the injured area.

21. A 19-year-old man was struck in the side of the head with a steel pipe during a gang altercation. Blood-tinged fluid is draining from the ears and bruising appears behind the ears. The most appropriate management for this patient includes

   a. elevating the lower extremities and providing immediate transport.

   b. applying 100% oxygen and packing the ear with sterile gauze pads.

   c. controlling the drainage from the ear and applying spinal immobilization.

   d. applying spinal immobilization and oxygen while monitoring the patient for vomiting.

22. Basic shock management consists of
   a. applying and inflating the PASG, applying oxygen, and providing warmth.
   b. elevating the lower extremities, applying and inflating the PASG, and applying oxygen.
   c. applying oxygen, elevating the upper body, and providing warmth.
   d. applying oxygen, elevating the lower extremities, and providing warmth.

23. Damaged small blood vessels beneath the skin following blunt trauma manifests as
   a. mottling.
   b. cyanosis.
   c. hematoma.
   d. ecchymosis.

24. When assessing a patient with a gunshot wound, you should routinely
   a. apply ice directly to the wound.
   b. determine why the patient was shot.
   c. look for the presence of an exit wound.
   d. evaluate the pulses proximal to the wound.

25. Which of the following signs would you expect to see in the early stages of shock?
   a. Hypotension
   b. Restlessness
   c. Thready pulses
   d. Unconsciousness

Subtest 4 Practice Exam: Medical

1. When caring for a patient with an emotional or behavioral crisis, your primary concern should be
   a. your and your partner's safety.
   b. providing safe transport to the hospital.
   c. gathering all of the patient's medications.
   d. obtaining a complete past psychiatric history.

2. Which of the following signs and symptoms are most characteristic of diabetic coma?
   a. Cool, clammy skin and a slow onset
   b. Cool, clammy skin and a rapid onset
   c. Warm, dry skin and a slow onset
   d. Warm, dry skin and a rapid onset

3. When assessing a conscious patient with a drug overdose, you should first ascertain
   a. the patient's weight in kilograms.
   b. the type of medication ingested.
   c. the time the medication was ingested.
   d. a history of other drugs ingested.

A ✓

4. The daughter of an elderly patient states that her mother is acting confused and talking incoherently. This nature of illness is most consistent with
   a. altered mental status.
   b. behavioral problems.
   c. cardiac compromise.
   d. diabetic complications.

A ✓

5. A 32-year-old man who was stung by a bee has generalized hives, facial swelling, and difficulty breathing. When he breathes, you hear audible stridor. What does this indicate?
   a. Swelling of the upper airway structures
   b. Swelling of the lower airway structures
   c. Narrowing of the two mainstem bronchi
   d. Narrowing of the bronchioles in the lungs

B ✓

6. A 28-year-old woman has severe lower quadrant abdominal pain. When assessing her abdomen, you should
   a. ask her where the pain is located and palpate that area first.
   b. ask her where the pain is located and palpate that area last.
   c. auscultate for bowel sounds for approximately 2 to 5 minutes.
   d. encourage the patient to lie supine with her legs fully extended.

A ✓

7. A 50-year-old woman who is awake and alert states that she has a severe migraine headache. When caring for her, you should avoid
   a. unnecessarily checking her pupils.
   b. transporting her in a supine position.
   c. dimming the lights in the ambulance.
   d. taking frequent blood pressure readings.

C ✓

8. Which of the following findings would be most significant during an assessment of a patient with a severe headache?
   a. Pain in both legs
   b. Chest discomfort
   c. Unilateral weakness
   d. Abdominal tenderness

D×A

9. A young woman reports significant weight loss over the last month, persistent fever, and night sweats. When you assess her, you note the presence of purplish lesions covering her trunk and upper extremities. You should suspect
   a. HIV/AIDS.
   b. tuberculosis.
   c. rheumatic fever.
   d. end-stage cancer.

B ✓

10. After having been bitten on the leg by a rattlesnake, a 45-year-old hiker complains of generalized weakness and shortness of breath. His blood pressure is 90/50 mm Hg, and his pulse rate is 120 beats/min. The most appropriate management of this patient includes
   a. oxygen, elevation of the affected part, ice packs.
   b. oxygen, lowering of the affected part, immobilization.
   c. oxygen, ice packs to the wound, immobilization.
   d. oxygen, proximal arterial constricting band, immobilization.

11. When you respond to a call, you find a 50-year-old woman with a history of epilepsy who is actively having a seizure. Care for this patient should focus primarily on
   a. frequent airway suctioning.
   b. ensuring effective ventilation.
   c. requesting an ALS ambulance.
   d. protecting the patient from injury.

12. When you arrive at a residence for a man who is "not acting right," you enter the house and notice a man sitting on his couch. Which of the following findings would be most indicative of an altered mental state?
   a. Medication bottles are present.
   b. The patient's eyes are closed.
   c. The patient appears to be tired.
   d. The patient has an abnormal speech pattern.

──────── **Questions 13 to 15 pertain to the following scenario:** ────────

You are called to a local park for a "man down." The temperature outside is approximately 95°. When you arrive, you are directed to the patient, a young man who is semiconscious. His skin is red, hot, and moist. You are told that the man had been drinking alcohol all day during a party.

13. Your first action in the management of this patient should be to
   a. ensure an open airway.
   b. move him to a cool area.
   c. administer 100% oxygen.
   d. initiate rapid cooling measures.

14. Based on the patient's initial presentation, you should suspect this patient has
   a. heatstroke.
   b. heat exhaustion.
   c. anaphylactic shock.
   d. a diabetic complication.

15. Body temperature is regulated by which of the following structures located within the brain?
   a. Cerebrum
   b. Cerebellum
   c. Hypothalamus
   d. Medulla oblongata

16. When caring for a patient with severe hypothermia who is in cardiac arrest, you should
   a. avoid using the AED.
   b. hyperventilate the patient.
   c. perform BLS and transport.
   d. perform rescue breathing only.

17. You are transporting a 30-year-old man who is experiencing an emotional crisis. The patient does not speak when you ask him questions. How should you respond to his unwillingness to speak?
  a. Remain silent until the patient speaks to you.
  b. Continually encourage the patient to talk to you.
  c. Tell the patient that you cannot help if he won't talk.
  d. Do not speak to the patient, even if he begins to speak to you.

18. Hypoxia-induced unconsciousness during a drowning or near-drowning episode is the result of
  a. laryngospasm.
  b. water in the lungs.
  c. cardiac arrhythmias.
  d. associated hypothermia.

19. In general, a frostbitten extremity should NOT be rewarmed if
  a. the part could refreeze after rewarming.
  b. a paramedic is not present to administer analgesia.
  c. you are unable to obtain water that is at least 120°.
  d. arrival at the emergency department will be delayed.

―――――― **Questions 20 to 22 pertain to the following scenario:** ――――――
You are called to an assisted living center where an attendant found a 76-year-old man unconscious. The patient had a recent hip replacement for which he is taking hydrocodone (Vicodin). During your initial assessment, you find that the patient is completely unresponsive. His respirations are 8 breaths/min and shallow and his heart rate is 40 beats/min.

20. On the basis of your initial assessment findings, your first course of action should be to
  a. apply 100% oxygen via a nonrebreathing mask.
  b. initiate positive pressure ventilations with a BVM device.
  c. request an ALS ambulance to respond to the scene.
  d. contact medical control for permission to give oral glucose.

21. With the patient's history in mind, as well as the type of medication that he is taking, what other abnormalities might you expect to find?
  a. Hypertension
  b. Dilated pupils
  c. Constricted pupils
  d. Increased tidal volume

22. Propoxyphene (Darvon) is categorized as what type of drug?
  a. Narcotic
  b. Barbiturate
  c. Amphetamine
  d. Benzodiazepine

_____ **23.** A 55-year-old woman with a history of insulin-dependant diabetes is found unconscious with rapid, shallow respirations. The patient's husband tells you that he does not know when his wife last took her insulin. Management of this patient should include
a. assisted ventilations and oral glucose.
b. assisted ventilations and rapid transport.
c. oral glucose and oxygen via nonrebreathing mask.
d. subcutaneous injection of insulin and 100% oxygen.

_____ **24.** When restraining a violent patient, you should make sure that
a. at least two EMT-Bs restrain the patient.
b. the patient is restrained using maximal force.
c. someone talks to the patient during the process.
d. consent for restraint has been obtained from a family member.

_____ **25.** Which of the following organs are contained within the right upper abdominal quadrant?
a. Liver and spleen
b. Liver and stomach
c. Liver and gallbladder
d. Stomach and gallbladder

Subtest 5 Practice Exam: Obstetrics and Pediatrics

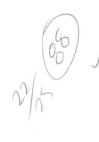

_____ **1.** Seizures in children most often are the result of
a. a life-threatening infection.
b. a temperature greater than 102°F.
c. an abrupt rise in body temperature.
d. an inflammatory process in the brain.

_____ **2.** After clearing the airway of a newborn who is not in distress, it is most important for you to
a. apply free-flow oxygen.
b. clamp and cut the cord.
c. keep the newborn warm.
d. obtain an APGAR score.

_____ **3.** You are caring for a 6-year-old child with a possible fractured left arm and have reason to believe that the child was abused. How should you manage this situation?
a. Inform the parents of your suspicions.
b. Call the police so the parents can be arrested.
c. Advise the parents that the child needs to be transported.
d. Transport the child to the hospital regardless of the parents' wishes.

At 0345, you receive a call for a woman in labor. Upon arriving at the scene, you are greeted by a very anxious man who tells you that his wife is having her baby "now." The man escorts you into the living room where a 25-year-old woman is lying on the couch in obvious pain.

4. The woman states that her contractions are occurring every 4 to 5 minutes and lasting approximately 30 seconds each. Which of the following questions would be most appropriate to ask at this point?
   a. Has your bag of waters broken yet?
   b. Have you had regular prenatal care?
   c. At how many weeks gestation are you?
   d. How many other children do you have?

5. Which of the following statements regarding crowning is true?
   a. Crowning represents the end of the second stage of labor.
   b. Crowning always occurs immediately after the amniotic sac has ruptured.
   c. It is safe to transport the patient during crowning if the hospital is close.
   d. Gentle pressure should be applied to the baby's head during crowning.

6. After determining that delivery is not imminent, you begin transport. While en route, the mother tells you that she feels the urge to push. You assess her and see the top of the baby's head bulging from the vagina. What is your most appropriate first action?
   a. Allow the head to deliver and check for the location of the cord.
   b. Advise your partner to stop the ambulance and assist with the delivery.
   c. Tell the mother to take short, quick breaths until you arrive at the hospital.
   d. Prepare the mother for an emergency delivery and open the obstetrics kit.

7. Upon assessing a newborn immediately after delivery, you note that the infant is breathing spontaneously and has a heart rate of 90 beats/min. What is the most appropriate initial management for this newborn?
   a. Begin positive pressure ventilations.
   b. Provide blow-by oxygen with oxygen tubing.
   c. Assess the newborn's skin condition and color.
   d. Start chest compressions and contact medical control.

8. Your assessment of a mother in active labor reveals that a limb is protruding from the vagina. Management of this condition should include
   a. positioning the mother in a semi-Fowler's position, administering oxygen, and providing transport.
   b. positioning the mother in a head-down position with her hips elevated, administering oxygen, and providing transport.
   c. applying gentle traction to the protruding limb to remove pressure of the fetus from the umbilical cord.
   d. giving the mother 100% oxygen and attempting to manipulate the protruding limb so that delivery can occur.

9. When you attempt to assess a 22-year-old woman who has been sexually assaulted, she orders you not to touch her. Your most appropriate initial action should be to
   a. ask the patient to sign a release form.
   b. ask a female EMT-B to attempt to assess the patient.
   c. explain to the patient that she must be examined.
   d. transport the patient without performing an assessment.

10. Which of the following techniques represents the most appropriate method of opening the airway of an infant with no suspected neck injury?
    a. Lift up the chin and hyperextend the neck.
    b. Tilt the head back without hyperextending the neck.
    c. Gently lift the chin while maintaining slight flexion of the neck.
    d. Perform the technique as you would for an older child or adult.

11. A 3-year-old child has a sudden onset of respiratory distress. The mother denies any recent illnesses or fever. You should suspect
    a. croup.
    b. epiglottitis.
    c. lower respiratory infection.
    d. foreign body airway obstruction.

12. Which of the following findings would indicate an altered mental status in a small child?
    a. Recognition of the parents
    b. Fright at the EMT-B's presence
    c. Lack of attention to the EMT-B's presence
    d. Consistent eye contact with the EMT-B

13. Which of the following parameters would be LEAST reliable when assessing the perfusion status of a 2-year-old child with possible shock?
    a. Distal capillary refill
    b. Systolic blood pressure
    c. Skin color and temperature
    d. Presence of peripheral pulses

14. Care for an alert 4-year-old child with a mild airway obstruction, who has respiratory distress, a strong cough, and normal skin color includes
    a. back blows, abdominal thrusts, transport.
    b. oxygen, avoiding agitation, transport.
    c. assisting ventilations, back blows, transport.
    d. chest thrusts, finger sweeps, transport.

15. You are called to a residence for a "sick" 5-year-old child. When you arrive and begin your assessment, you note that the child is unconscious with a respiratory rate of 8 breaths/min and a heart rate of 50 beats/min. Management of this child should consist of
    a. 100% oxygen via a nonrebreathing mask and rapid transport.
    b. positive pressure ventilations with a BVM device and rapid transport.
    c. chest compressions, artificial ventilations, and rapid transport.
    d. back blows and chest thrusts while attempting artificial ventilations.

16. Following delivery of a newborn, the 21-year-old mother is experiencing mild vaginal bleeding. You note that her heart rate has increased from 90 to 120 beats/min and she is diaphoretic. Management should include
a. oxygen, uterine massage, and transport.
b. oxygen, placement on the left side, and transport.
c. oxygen, treatment for shock, and uterus massage during transport.
d. oxygen, internal vaginal pads, and treatment of shock during transport.

17. While performing a visual inspection of a 30-year-old woman in active labor, you can see the umbilical cord at the vaginal opening. After providing high concentration oxygen, you should next
a. massage the uterus to facilitate delivery of the fetus.
b. relieve pressure from the cord with your gloved fingers.
c. place the mother on her left side and provide rapid transport.
d. elevate the mother's lower extremities and provide immediate transport.

18. A 34-year-old woman, who is 36 weeks pregnant, is having a seizure. After you protect her airway and ensure adequate ventilation, you should transport her
a. on her left side.
b. in the prone position.
c. in the supine position.
d. in a semisitting position.

19. A 7-year-old child has an altered mental status, high fever, and a generalized rash. You perform your assessment and initiate oxygen therapy. En route to the hospital, you should be most alert for
a. vomiting.
b. seizures.
c. combativeness.
d. respiratory distress.

20. Which of the following is the most common cause of shock (hypoperfusion) in infants and children?
a. Infection
b. Cardiac failure
c. Accidental poisoning
d. Severe allergic reaction

21. Which of the following signs or symptoms is more common in children than adults following head trauma?
a. Nausea and vomiting
b. Altered mental status
c. Tachycardia and diaphoresis
d. Changes in pupillary reaction

22. A 4-year-old girl fell from a third-story window and landed on her head. She is semiconscious with slow, irregular breathing and bleeding from her mouth. After performing a jaw-thrust maneuver with simultaneous stabilization of her head, you should
a. suction the oropharynx.
b. insert a nasopharyngeal airway.
c. initiate positive pressure ventilations.
d. administer oxygen via nonrebreathing mask.

23. Which of the following statements regarding 2-rescuer child CPR is correct?
  a. The chest should not be allowed to fully recoil in between compressions as this may impede venous return
  b. Compress the chest with one or two hands to a depth equal to one-half to one third the diameter of the chest
  c. The chest should be compressed with one hand and a compression to ventilation ratio of 30:2 should be delivered
  d. A compression to ventilation ratio of 15:2 should be delivered without pauses in compressions to deliver ventilations

24. General guidelines when assessing a 2-year-old child with abdominal pain and adequate perfusion include
  a. examining the child in the parent's arms.
  b. palpating the painful area of the abdomen first.
  c. placing the child supine and palpating the abdomen.
  d. separating the child from the parent to ensure a reliable examination.

25. You are managing a 10-month-old infant who has had severe diarrhea and vomiting for 3 days and is now showing signs of shock. You have initiated supplemental oxygen therapy and elevated the lower extremities. En route to the hospital, you note that the child's work of breathing has increased. What must you do first?
  a. Lower the extremities and reassess the child.
  b. Begin positive pressure ventilations and reassess the child.
  c. Place a nasopharyngeal airway and increase the oxygen flow.
  d. Listen to the lungs with a stethoscope for abnormal breath sounds.

Subtest 6 Practice Exam: Operations

1. The safest ambulance driver is one who
  a. is physically fit.
  b. has a positive attitude.
  c. drives with due regard.
  d. drives with lights and siren.

2. You are called to treat a 25-year-old man who is alert and having difficulty breathing. After making contact with your patient, he extends his arm out to allow you to take his blood pressure. This is an example of
  a. actual consent.
  b. informed consent.
  c. implied consent.
  d. formal consent.

3. You are providing care to a male patient at the scene of a shooting. The police are at the scene collecting evidence. Your actions should include
  a. limiting your care to the initial assessment.
  b. beginning care when the police authorize you to.
  c. beginning immediate care as you would with any other patient.
  d. providing care to the patient while manipulating the scene minimally.

C ✓

4. Which of the following statements regarding the use of an escort vehicle when en route to an emergency call is true?
   a. An escort vehicle will allow you to arrive at the scene quicker.
   b. To avoid getting separated from the escort vehicle, you should closely follow it.
   c. An escort vehicle should be used only if you are unfamiliar with the patient's location.
   d. With an escort vehicle, the risk of an accident at an intersection is reduced significantly.

B ✓

5. You arrive at the scene of a fall where you encounter a male patient who fell approximately 30′ and landed on his head. He is unconscious with an open head injury and exposed brain matter. Upon identifying this patient as an organ donor, you should
   a. request authorization from medical control not to initiate care.
   b. manage the patient aggressively and provide rapid transport.
   c. recognize that the patient's injuries disqualify him as an organ donor.
   d. provide supportive care only because the patient likely will not survive.

C

6. You are giving a presentation to a group of laypeople on the importance of calling EMS immediately for cardiac arrest patients. What point should you emphasize the most?
   a. Laypeople are incapable of providing adequate CPR.
   b. Rapid transport significantly reduces patient mortality.
   c. CPR and defibrillation are key factors in patient survival.
   d. Cardiac drug therapy is the most important EMS treatment.

C

7. As an EMT-Basic, your primary responsibility is to
   a. provide competent patient care.
   b. ensure the safety of your partner.
   c. keep yourself as safe as possible.
   d. transport all patients to the hospital.

D ✓

8. You arrive at the scene of a traffic accident in which multiple vehicles are involved. You see at least two patients who appear to be unconscious. Your first action should be to
   a. begin triaging the patients.
   b. begin immediate patient care.
   c. notify medical control for advice.
   d. request an additional ambulance.

B A

9. When providing care to multiple patients at the scene of a mass-casualty incident, your goal should remain focused on
   a. transporting patients to the hospital.
   b. immobilizing all patients at the scene.
   c. initiating CPR for those in cardiac arrest.
   d. keeping all bystanders at a safe distance.

10. Immediately upon leaving the scene with a patient, you should
   a. contact medical control.
   b. notify the receiving facility.
   c. advise dispatch of your status.
   d. conduct a detailed examination.

11. When you arrive at a mass-casualty incident at which other ambulances already
have arrived, you should first
a. repeat the triage process.
b. report to the incident commander.
c. initiate care for the most critically injured patients.
d. obtain information from the fire service commander.

12. During the triage process, which of the following injuries or conditions would
classify a patient as a high priority?
a. Pulselessness and apnea
b. Unilateral femur fracture and tachycardia
c. Partial-thickness burns with no respiratory difficulty
d. A large avulsion to the arm and an altered mental status

13. The role of triage officer at a mass-casualty incident should be assumed by the
a. most knowledgeable EMS provider.
b. EMS provider with the most years of experience.
c. first EMS provider who is willing to perform the task.
d. EMS medical director via telephone communication.

14. The information that would be of LEAST pertinence when educating the public
on injury prevention is
a. how to provide rescue breathing.
b. the proper usage of child safety seats.
c. building a childproof fence around a pool.
d. teaching children to wear bicycle helmets.

15. You are called to a residence for a woman in cardiac arrest. As you are initiating
CPR, the patient's husband presents you with an unsigned document that states
"do not resuscitate." Your most appropriate action in this case should be to
a. stop all resuscitative efforts in accordance with the document.
b. stop CPR until the document can be validated by a physician.
c. continue CPR until you have contacted medical control for guidance.
d. contact medical control prior to beginning any resuscitation measures.

16. According to the United States Department of Transportation's EMT-Basic
National Standard Curriculum, minimum staffing for a basic life support
ambulance includes
a. an EMT-Basic who functions as the driver.
b. at least one EMT-Basic in the patient compartment.
c. at least two EMT-Basics in the patient compartment.
d. a minimum of two EMT-Basics in the ambulance.

17. The ultimate goal of any EMS quality improvement program should be to
a. deliver a consistently high standard of care to all patients who are
encountered.
b. make sure that all personnel receive an adequate number of continuing
education credits.
c. provide EMS protocols to all EMTs and hold them accountable when
protocols are not adhered to.
d. provide recognition to all EMTs who have demonstrated consistency in
providing competent patient care.

18. You are caring for a 6-year-old child with a swollen, painful deformity to the left forearm. As you communicate with the parents of this child, you should
a. ask them repeatedly how the child was injured.
b. use appropriate medical terminology at all times.
c. make sure that they remain aware of what you are doing.
d. tell them that the child will be transported to the hospital.

19. Following a call in which a 6-week-old infant in cardiac arrest did not survive, your partner is exhibiting significant anxiety and irritability. How can you most effectively help her?
a. Allow her to voice her feelings to you.
b. Tell her that she needs psychiatric help.
c. Tell her to go home and get 12 hours of sleep.
d. Report her behavior to the medical director.

20. When is it most appropriate to complete your prehospital care report for a critically ill patient?
a. During the initial assessment phase
b. During the ongoing assessment phase
c. As soon as all patient care activities are completed
d. After the ambulance has been restocked at the station

21. Which of the following scene size-up findings is LEAST suggestive of an unsafe environment?
a. A large man standing in his yard awaiting your arrival
b. Liquid draining from a car that struck a telephone pole
c. Screaming and yelling coming from inside a residence
d. The sound of breaking glass as you approach a residence

22. Proper body mechanics when lifting and moving a patient include
a. maintaining a slight curvature of your back.
b. using the muscles of your lower back to lift.
c. keeping the weight as close to you as possible.
d. twisting at the waist when moving a patient around a corner.

23. The immobilization device most appropriate to use for a patient with multiple injuries and unstable vital signs is a
a. scoop immobilization device.
b. vest-style immobilization device.
c. short spine board immobilization device.
d. long spine board immobilization device.

24. Medical control has ordered you to administer one tube of oral glucose to your patient suspected of having hypoglycemia. Immediately after receiving this order, you should
a. document the order on the prehospital care report.
b. administer the medication and reassess the patient.
c. ask medical control to repeat the order word for word.
d. repeat the order back to medical control word for word.

_____ **25.** While caring for a critically injured patient, you remove blood-soaked clothing in order to manage injuries. You should dispose of the clothing by
  a. leaving it at the scene.
  b. leaving it at the hospital.
  c. placing it in a biohazard bag.
  d. placing it in the ambulance trash can.

Practice Final Examination

_____ **1.** Snoring respirations are most rapidly managed by
  a. suctioning the oropharynx.
  b. initiating assisted ventilations.
  c. correctly positioning the head.
  d. inserting an oropharyngeal airway.

_____ **2.** Which of the following patients would be most in need of a rapid trauma assessment?
  a. An awake and alert 19-year-old man with a small caliber gunshot wound to the abdomen
  b. A conscious 25-year-old woman who fell 12′ from a roof and landed on her side
  c. A 43-year-old woman with a unilaterally swollen, painful deformity of the femur
  d. A 60-year-old man who fell from a standing position and has an abrasion on his cheek

_____ **3.** Which of the following bones is affected with a swollen, painful deformity to the lateral bone of the left forearm?
  a. Ulna
  b. Radius
  c. Clavicle
  d. Humerus

_____ **4.** During your assessment of a 34-year-old man with a gunshot wound to the chest, you note that his skin is pale. This finding is most likely caused by
  a. a critically low blood pressure.
  b. increased blood flow to the skin.
  c. decreased blood flow to the skin.
  d. peripheral dilation of the vasculature.

_____ **5.** An 80-year-old woman has pain in the right upper quadrant of her abdomen and a yellowish tinge to her skin. You should suspect dysfunction of the
  a. liver.
  b. spleen.
  c. pancreas.
  d. gallbladder.

_____ **6.** Which of the following situations is an example of abandonment?
  a. An EMT-Paramedic gives a verbal report to an emergency nurse.
  b. An EMT-Intermediate assumes patient care from an EMT-Basic.
  c. An EMT-Basic transfers care of a patient to an EMT-Paramedic.
  d. A first responder assumes patient care from an EMT-Intermediate.

_____ **7.** Which artery should you palpate when assessing for a pulse in an unresponsive 6-month-old patient?
a. Radial
b. Carotid
c. Femoral
d. Brachial

_____ **8.** During the initial assessment of a trauma patient, you note massive facial injuries, weak radial pulses, and clammy skin. What should be your most immediate concern?
a. Potential obstruction of the airway
b. Internal bleeding and severe shock
c. Applying 100% supplemental oxygen
d. Providing rapid transport to a trauma center

_____ **9.** You are called to treat a male patient who overdosed on heroin and is unconscious with shallow breathing and cyanosis to the face. The patient suddenly begins to vomit. What should you do first?
a. Suction the oropharynx.
b. Turn the patient onto his side.
c. Insert an oropharyngeal airway.
d. Assist ventilations with 100% oxygen.

_____ **10.** The scene size-up includes all of the following components, EXCEPT
a. determining scene safety.
b. applying personal protective gear.
c. assessing the need for assistance.
d. evaluating the mechanism of injury.

_____ **11.** In which of the following patients would an oropharyngeal airway be indicated?
a. Any patient suspected of having hypoxia
b. A semiconscious patient with an intact gag reflex
c. A semiconscious patient who took an overdose of propoxyphene
d. An unconscious patient with fluid drainage from the ears

_____ **12.** Upon arriving at the scene of a multiple vehicle crash, you can see that at least two patients have been ejected from their vehicles. What should you do next?
a. Begin triage.
b. Treat the most critical patient first.
c. Gather all of the patients together.
d. Call for at least one more ambulance.

_____ **13.** A 75-year-old man has generalized weakness and chest pain. He has a bottle of prescribed nitroglycerin, and he states that he has not taken any of his medication. After initiating oxygen therapy, you should next
a. apply the AED and prepare the patient for immediate transport.
b. perform a detailed physical examination to locate any other problems.
c. contact medical control for permission to assist the patient with his nitroglycerin.
d. complete a focused physical examination, including obtaining baseline vital signs.

_____ **14.** Which of the following organs is not part of the endocrine system?
  a. Thyroid
  b. Pituitary
  c. Pancreas
  d. Gallbladder

_____ **15.** Which of the following injuries or conditions should be managed first?
  a. Fluid drainage from both ears
  b. Bleeding within the oral cavity
  c. A large open abdominal wound
  d. Bilateral fractures of the femurs

_____ **16.** You arrive at a residence where you find a man lying unconscious in his front yard. There were no witnesses to the event that caused the unconsciousness. In assessing this man, you must assume that he
  a. has sustained an injury.
  b. is having a heart attack.
  c. is having a diabetic reaction.
  d. is having a heat-related emergency.

_____ **17.** When is the best time to perform a detailed physical examination?
  a. While en route to the hospital
  b. After all life threats have been ruled out
  c. Immediately after taking baseline vital signs
  d. Following the initial assessment of a trauma patient

_____ **18.** Which of the following conditions would most likely cause flushed skin?
  a. Shock
  b. Hypoxia
  c. Exposure to heat
  d. Low blood pressure

_____ **19.** During the rapid trauma assessment of a patient with multiple injuries, you expose the chest and find an open wound with blood bubbling from it. What should you do next?
  a. Apply 100% supplemental oxygen.
  b. Provide rapid transport to the hospital.
  c. Prevent air from entering the wound.
  d. Place a porous dressing over the wound.

_____ **20.** You are called to a local park for a 7-year-old boy with respiratory distress. During your assessment, you find that the patient is wheezing and has widespread hives and facial edema. What should you suspect has occurred?
  a. Heat emergency
  b. Allergic reaction
  c. Acute asthma attack
  d. Exposure to a poisonous plant

_____ **21.** A common side effect of nitroglycerin is
  a. nausea.
  b. headache.
  c. hypertension.
  d. chest discomfort.

_____ **22.** As you assess a 56-year-old man, you note that he is pulseless and apneic. As your partner gets the AED from the ambulance, you should
  a. obtain a medical history from the wife.
  b. place the patient in the recovery position.
  c. perform CPR until the AED is ready to use.
  d. conduct a detailed examination of the patient.

_____ **23.** Prescribed inhalers, such as albuterol (Ventolin), relieve respiratory distress by
  a. constricting the bronchioles in the lungs.
  b. contracting the smaller airways in the lungs.
  c. relaxing the smooth muscle of the bronchioles.
  d. dilating the large mainstem bronchi of the airway.

_____ **24.** In a patient with cardiac compromise, you would be LEAST likely to encounter
  a. anxiety.
  b. dyspnea.
  c. headache.
  d. chest pain.

_____ **25.** When monitoring a patient with a head injury, the most reliable indicator of his or her condition is the
  a. pupillary reaction.
  b. level of consciousness.
  c. systolic blood pressure.
  d. rate and depth of breathing.

_____ **26.** A 56-year-old man with a history of cardiac problems reports pain in the upper midabdominal area. This region of the abdomen is called the
  a. peritoneum.
  b. epigastrium.
  c. mediastinum.
  d. retroperitoneum.

_____ **27.** Which of the following mechanisms cause respiratory and circulatory collapse during anaphylactic shock?
  a. Bronchodilation and vasodilation
  b. Bronchodilation and vasoconstriction
  c. Bronchoconstriction and vasodilation
  d. Bronchoconstriction and vasoconstriction

_____ **28.** In the patient with diabetes, hypoglycemia typically presents with
  a. dry skin and a slow onset.
  b. dry skin and a rapid onset.
  c. clammy skin and a slow onset.
  d. clammy skin and a rapid onset.

_____ **29.** Which of the following signs would LEAST suggest a diabetic emergency?
   a. Bradycardia
   b. Tachycardia
   c. Combativeness
   d. Fruity breath odor

_____ **30.** Which of the following patients would be at most risk for suicide?
   a. A woman who quit her job for one that pays more
   b. A man who is in the midst of losing a significant relationship
   c. A man who is planning a family trip, but gets called away to work
   d. An EMT who saved a drowning child and receives a lot of media attention

_____ **31.** A middle-aged woman has acute shortness of breath and respirations of 30 breaths/min. How should you first manage this patient?
   a. Assess respiratory quality.
   b. Begin assisting ventilations.
   c. Apply supplemental oxygen.
   d. Perform a detailed examination.

_____ **32.** To obtain the most reliable assessment of a patient's tidal volume, you should
   a. assess for retractions.
   b. listen for airway noises.
   c. count the respiratory rate.
   d. look at the rise of the chest.

_____ **33.** As you are performing CPR on an elderly man, his wife presents you with a "do not resuscitate" order. Your most appropriate course of action is to
   a. ignore the document and continue CPR.
   b. comply with the document and stop CPR.
   c. continue CPR until medical control is notified.
   d. withhold CPR until medical control validates the order.

_____ **34.** A 5-year-old boy complains of pain to the right lower quadrant of his abdomen. Correct assessment of this child's abdomen includes
   a. avoiding palpation of the abdomen.
   b. palpating the left upper quadrant first.
   c. auscultating bowel sounds for 2 minutes.
   d. palpating the right lower quadrant first.

_____ **35.** In most states, the EMT-Basic is required to report which of the following occurrences?
   a. Animal bite
   b. Drug overdose
   c. Injury to a minor
   d. Motor vehicle crash

_____ **36.** A set of regulations and ethical considerations that define the extent or limits of an EMT-Basic's job is called
   a. a duty to act.
   b. confidentiality.
   c. scope of practice.
   d. the Medical Practices Act.

_____ **37.** A 9-year-old girl was struck by a car while she was crossing the street and is displaying signs of shock. During your assessment, you note a large contusion over the left upper quadrant of her abdomen. Which of the following organs has most likely been injured?
a. Liver
b. Kidney
c. Spleen
d. Pancreas

_____ **38.** The automated external defibrillator (AED) should NOT be used in patients who
a. are between 1 and 8 years of age.
b. experienced a witnessed cardiac arrest.
c. are apneic and have a weak carotid pulse.
d. have a nitroglycerin patch applied to the skin.

_____ **39.** As you step out of the ambulance at the scene of a nighttime motor vehicle crash on the highway, your immediate concern should be
a. oncoming traffic.
b. whether the car will catch on fire.
c. placing safety flares by the ambulance.
d. quick assessment of the patients in the car.

_____ **40.** Which of the following actions should be carried out during the initial assessment of an unconscious patient?
a. Assessing the skin
b. Palpating the cranium
c. Auscultating the lungs
d. Obtaining a blood pressure

—————— **Questions 41 to 43 pertain to the following scenario:**——————
You arrive at the scene shortly after a 55-year-old man collapsed. Two bystanders are performing CPR. The man's wife states the he had cardiac by-pass surgery approximately 6 months earlier. There are no signs of trauma.

_____ **41.** Your first action in the management of this patient should be to
a. attach an AED and analyze the cardiac rhythm.
b. check the effectiveness of the CPR in progress.
c. insert an oropharyngeal airway and continue CPR.
d. stop CPR so you can assess pulse and breathing.

_____ **42.** Cardiac arrest in the adult population is most often the result of
a. an acute stroke.
b. respiratory failure.
c. cardiac arrhythmias.
d. myocardial infarction.

_____ **43.** After you attach the AED and analyze this patient's heart rhythm, the machine states, "shock advised." What cardiac rhythm is the patient most likely in?
a. Asystole
b. Ventricular fibrillation
c. Ventricular tachycardia
d. Pulseless electrical activity

_____ **44.** Immediately upon delivery of a newborn's head, you should first
  a. dry the face.
  b. cover the eyes.
  c. suction the nose.
  d. suction the mouth.

_____ **45.** You assess a newborn with cyanosis to the chest and face and a heart rate of 90 beats/min. What should you do next?
  a. Resuction the mouth.
  b. Briskly dry off the infant.
  c. Begin chest compressions.
  d. Begin artificial ventilations.

_____ **46.** An EMT-B's failure to obtain consent to treat a patient could result in allegations of
  a. battery.
  b. negligence.
  c. abandonment.
  d. breach of duty.

_____ **47.** Which of the following describes the MOST appropriate method of performing chest compressions on an adult patient in cardiac arrest?
  a. Compress the chest to a depth of 1 ½" to 2", allow full recoil of the chest after each compression, minimize interruptions in chest compressions
  b. Allow full recoil of the chest after each compression, compress the chest to a depth of 2", deliver compressions at a rate of at least 80/min
  c. Do not interrupt chest compressions for any reason, compress the chest to a depth of 1 ½" to 2", allow partial recoil of the chest after each compression
  d. Minimize interruptions in chest compressions, provide 70% compression time and 30% relaxation time, deliver compressions at a rate of 100/min

_____ **48.** Prevention of cardiac arrest in infants and small children should focus primarily on
  a. keeping the child warm.
  b. avoiding upsetting the child.
  c. providing immediate transport.
  d. providing airway management.

_____ **49.** You are managing a conscious patient who you believe is having an acute ischemic stroke. After administering oxygen, your next priority should include
  a. providing prompt transport for possible fibrinolytic therapy.
  b. determining whether the patient has prescribed nitroglycerin.
  c. closely monitoring the blood pressure every 15 to 20 minutes.
  d. completing a detailed physical examination before providing transport.

_____ **50.** Which of the following patients with diabetes should receive oral glucose?
  a. A confused patient who has cool, clammy skin
  b. A confused patient who has suspected hyperglycemia
  c. A semiconscious patient with pale skin
  d. An unconscious patient who took too much insulin

_____ **51.** During a bar fight, a 22-year-old man was stabbed in the chest with a large knife. The patient is pulseless and apneic, and the knife is impaled in the center of his chest. Management should include
  a. stabilizing the knife, starting CPR, and providing rapid transport.
  b. stabilizing the knife, applying an occlusive dressing, and providing rapid transport.
  c. removing the knife, starting CPR, and providing rapid transport.
  d. removing the knife, applying an occlusive dressing, and providing rapid transport.

_____ **52.** In which of the following patients would nitroglycerin be contraindicated?
  a. 41-year-old male with crushing chest pressure, a blood pressure of 160/90 mm Hg, and severe nausea
  b. 53-year-old male with chest discomfort, diaphoresis, a blood pressure of 146/66 mm Hg, and regular use of Cialis
  c. 58-year-old male with chest pain radiating to the left arm, a blood pressure of 130/64 mm Hg, and prescribed Tegretol
  d. 66-year-old female with chest pressure of 6 hours' duration, lightheadedness, and a blood pressure of 110/58 mm Hg

_____ **53.** Firefighters have rescued a man from his burning house. He is conscious and in considerable respiratory distress. He has a brassy cough and singed nasal hairs. The most immediate threat to this patient's life is
  a. hypothermia.
  b. severe burns.
  c. severe infection.
  d. closure of the airway.

_____ **54.** You respond to a call for a shooting at a local bar. You arrive at the scene and find a young man sitting against the wall, screaming in pain, with bright red blood spurting from a wound near his groin. What should you do first?
  a. Ensure an open airway.
  b. Administer 100% oxygen.
  c. Apply pressure to the wound.
  d. Transport the patient at once.

_____ **55.** Patients with closed head injuries often have pupillary changes and
  a. paralysis.
  b. paresthesia.
  c. hypertension.
  d. tachycardia.

_____ **56.** When assessing a patient with a reduction in tidal volume, you would expect the respirations to be
  a. deep.
  b. labored.
  c. shallow.
  d. dyspneic.

_____ **57.** Prior to applying a nonrebreathing mask on a patient with difficulty breathing, you should
   a. set the flow rate to no more than 10 L/min.
   b. prefill the reservoir bag to ensure delivery of 100% oxygen.
   c. insert a nasopharyngeal airway to maintain airway patency.
   d. perform a complete physical examination to determine the degree of hypoxia.

_____ **58.** A 60-year-old woman is experiencing severe respiratory distress. When you ask her a question, she can only say two words at a time. You should manage this patient by
   a. inserting a nasopharyngeal airway.
   b. providing positive pressure ventilations.
   c. applying a nasal cannula set at 2 to 6 L/min.
   d. applying a nonrebreathing mask set at 15 L/min.

_____ **59.** The most effective method for determining whether you are providing adequate artificial ventilation is
   a. assessing the chest for adequate rise.
   b. assessing the pulse for an improving heart rate.
   c. checking the pupils for increased reactivity.
   d. checking the skin for improvement of cyanosis.

_____ **60.** You are administering oxygen to a woman with asthma who took two puffs of her prescribed inhaler without relief prior to your arrival. Your next action should be to
   a. contact medical control for further advice.
   b. administer one more puff from the inhaler.
   c. provide immediate transport to the hospital.
   d. confirm that her inhaler is prescribed to her.

_____ **61.** Unconsciousness, shallow breathing, and constricted pupils are most indicative of what type of drug overdose?
   a. Narcotic
   b. Marijuana
   c. Barbiturate
   d. Amphetamine

_____ **62.** When dealing with an emotionally disturbed patient, you should be concerned with
   a. providing safe transport.
   b. whether the patient could harm you.
   c. obtaining a complete medical history.
   d. gathering all of the patient's medications.

_____ **63.** During your initial assessment of an unconscious adult patient, you find the patient is apneic. You should next
   a. assess for a carotid pulse.
   b. begin chest compressions.
   c. deliver two rescue breaths.
   d. place an oropharyngeal airway.

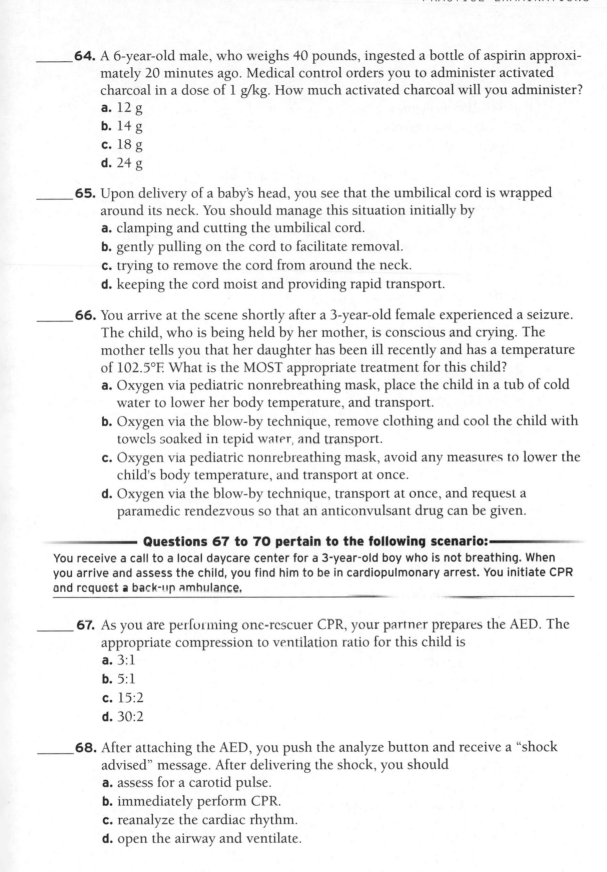

_____ **64.** A 6-year-old male, who weighs 40 pounds, ingested a bottle of aspirin approximately 20 minutes ago. Medical control orders you to administer activated charcoal in a dose of 1 g/kg. How much activated charcoal will you administer?
   a. 12 g
   b. 14 g
   c. 18 g
   d. 24 g

_____ **65.** Upon delivery of a baby's head, you see that the umbilical cord is wrapped around its neck. You should manage this situation initially by
   a. clamping and cutting the umbilical cord.
   b. gently pulling on the cord to facilitate removal.
   c. trying to remove the cord from around the neck.
   d. keeping the cord moist and providing rapid transport.

_____ **66.** You arrive at the scene shortly after a 3-year-old female experienced a seizure. The child, who is being held by her mother, is conscious and crying. The mother tells you that her daughter has been ill recently and has a temperature of 102.5°F. What is the MOST appropriate treatment for this child?
   a. Oxygen via pediatric nonrebreathing mask, place the child in a tub of cold water to lower her body temperature, and transport.
   b. Oxygen via the blow-by technique, remove clothing and cool the child with towels soaked in tepid water, and transport.
   c. Oxygen via pediatric nonrebreathing mask, avoid any measures to lower the child's body temperature, and transport at once.
   d. Oxygen via the blow-by technique, transport at once, and request a paramedic rendezvous so that an anticonvulsant drug can be given.

────────── **Questions 67 to 70 pertain to the following scenario:** ──────────
You receive a call to a local daycare center for a 3-year-old boy who is not breathing. When you arrive and assess the child, you find him to be in cardiopulmonary arrest. You initiate CPR and request a back-up ambulance.

_____ **67.** As you are performing one-rescuer CPR, your partner prepares the AED. The appropriate compression to ventilation ratio for this child is
   a. 3:1
   b. 5:1
   c. 15:2
   d. 30:2

_____ **68.** After attaching the AED, you push the analyze button and receive a "shock advised" message. After delivering the shock, you should
   a. assess for a carotid pulse.
   b. immediately perform CPR.
   c. reanalyze the cardiac rhythm.
   d. open the airway and ventilate.

_____ **69.** A paramedic unit arrives at the scene to provide assistance. After one of the paramedics intubates the child, you should deliver ventilations at a rate of
a. 6 to 8 breaths/min.
b. 8 to 10 breaths/min.
c. 10 to 12 breaths/min.
d. 12 to 20 breaths/min.

_____ **70.** In infants and children, the most detrimental effect of gastric distention is
a. increased ease of ventilations.
b. decreased ventilatory volume.
c. acute rupture of the diaphragm.
d. less effective chest compressions.

_____ **71.** Which of the following parameters would be most reliable as an indicator of perfusion in a 1-year-old child?
a. Heart rate
b. Capillary refill
c. Blood pressure
d. Respiratory rate

_____ **72.** While managing a patient with acute shortness of breath, you prepare and apply a nonrebreathing mask set at 12 L/min. The patient pulls the mask away from his face, stating that it is smothering him. You should next
a. increase the oxygen flow and reapply the mask.
b. securely tape the oxygen mask to the patient's face.
c. reassure the patient and apply a nasal cannula instead.
d. inform the patient that refusing oxygen might result in his death.

_____ **73.** Signs of inadequate breathing in an unconscious patient include
a. a fast heart rate.
b. warm, moist skin.
c. equal breath sounds.
d. a rapid respiratory rate.

_____ **74.** Initial attempts at providing artificial ventilation should be accomplished using
a. the one-person bag-valve-mask technique.
b. the two-person bag-valve-mask technique.
c. a pocket mask with supplemental oxygen.
d. a flow-restricted oxygen-powered ventilation device.

_____ **75.** The most effective means of preventing the spread of disease is
a. effective handwashing.
b. up-to-date immunizations.
c. wearing gloves with all patients.
d. wearing a mask with all patients.

_____ **76.** You have completed your prehospital care report and left a copy at the hospital when you realize that you forgot to document a pertinent finding on the front of the report. Your most appropriate action would be to
  a. attach an addendum to the original run report.
  b. write the information on the original run report.
  c. complete a new run report and add the information.
  d. take no action and report the event to your supervisor.

_____ **77.** An awake and alert 92-year-old woman with chest pain is refusing EMS treatment and transport to the hospital. Her family insists that you transport her. This situation is most appropriately managed by
  a. transporting the patient as the family wishes.
  b. advising the patient of the risks of refusing care.
  c. obtaining a signed refusal from a family member.
  d. transporting the patient as you explain your actions.

_____ **78.** At the scene of a mass-casualty incident, you notice a bystander who is clearly emotionally upset. An appropriate action to take would be to
  a. tell the bystander to leave the scene at once.
  b. have the bystander assist you with patient care.
  c. notify the police and have the bystander removed.
  d. assign the bystander a simple, non-patient-care task.

_____ **79.** Which of the following situations would necessitate treatment using implied consent?
  a. A 16-year-old pregnant girl with an isolated extremity injury
  b. An 18-year-old man who is now alert after receiving oral glucose
  c. A 25-year-old man who is restless and has severe chest pain and diaphoresis
  d. A 65-year-old man who is semiconscious and suspected of having a severe stroke

_____ **80.** Which of the following patients would MOST likely present with atypical signs and symptoms of acute myocardial infarction?
  a. 72-year-old female with diabetes and hypertension.
  b. 64-year-old male with renal disease and depression.
  c. 59 year-old male with alcoholism and angina pectoris.
  d. 55-year-old female with COPD and frequent infections.

_____ **81.** While assessing a patient with chest pain, you note that the patient's pulse is irregular. This most likely indicates
  a. acute myocardial infarction or angina pectoris.
  b. a dysfunction in the left side of the patient's heart.
  c. high blood pressure that is increasing cardiac workload.
  d. abnormalities in the heart's electrical conduction system.

_____ **82.** While a man was using a chainsaw to trim branches from a tree, it slipped and caused a large laceration to his left forearm. Bright red blood is spurting from the wound. The patient is conscious, alert, and talking. You should first
    a. open the patient's airway.
    b. control the active bleeding.
    c. apply supplemental oxygen.
    d. thoroughly cleanse the wound.

_____ **83.** After an initial attempt to ventilate a patient fails, you reposition the patient's head and reattempt ventilation without success. You should next
    a. assess for a carotid pulse and initiate CPR if necessary.
    b. use a flow-restricted oxygen-powered ventilation device.
    c. initiate airway obstruction removal techniques and provide transport.
    d. continue to reposition the patient's head at the scene until you are able to secure a patent airway.

_____ **84.** A 40-year-old patient sustained full-thickness burns to the entire head, anterior chest, and both anterior upper extremities. Using the adult Rule of Nines, what percentage of the patient's body surface area has been burned?
    a. 18%
    b. 27%
    c. 36%
    d. 45%

_____ **85.** When assessing a patient with a complaint of chest pain, which of the following questions would you ask to assess the "R" in OPQRST?
    a. Did the pain begin suddenly or gradually?
    b. What were you doing when the pain began?
    c. Is there anything that makes the pain worse?
    d. Is the pain in one place or does it move around?

_____ **86.** Which of the following describes the most correct method for inserting a nasopharyngeal airway?
    a. Insert the device with the bevel facing the septum.
    b. Insert the device with the bevel facing the lateral aspect of the nose.
    c. Rotate the device as you insert it into the right nostril.
    d. Apply firm, gentle pressure if you meet resistance during insertion.

_____ **87.** Which vital sign is the best indicator of cardiac output during the initial assessment?
    a. Pulse rate and quality
    b. Systolic blood pressure
    c. Quality of the respirations
    d. Condition and color of the skin

_____ **88.** After assisting a patient with her epinephrine auto-injector, you should dispose of the device by
    a. giving it to the patient to have it refilled.
    b. placing the device in a red biohazard bag.
    c. placing the device in a puncture proof container.
    d. replacing the cover and putting it in a trash can.

_____ **89.** Which of the following assessment findings would most suggest a systemic reaction following ingestion of a poison?
  a. Nausea and vomiting
  b. Burns around the mouth
  c. Tachycardia and hypotension
  d. Difficulty swallowing and burning in the mouth

_____ **90.** You are at the scene where a man panicked while swimming in a small lake. As you attempt to rescue this patient, you should first
  a. throw a rope to the patient.
  b. row a small raft to the patient.
  c. swim to the patient to rescue him.
  d. attempt to grab the patient with a stick.

_____ **91.** After removing a patient from the water, your assessment reveals that the patient is breathing inadequately and is continuously regurgitating large quantities of water. You should manage this patient by
  a. alternating suctioning with artificial ventilations.
  b. performing abdominal thrusts to remove the water.
  c. placing the patient on the side and pressing on the abdomen.
  d. initiating artificial ventilations after the patient stops regurgitating.

_____ **92.** Your first action in managing a patient with an altered mental status should be to
  a. give the patient oral glucose.
  b. administer 100% supplemental oxygen.
  c. make sure that the patient is breathing adequately.
  d. try to determine the cause of the altered mental status.

_____ **93.** Management of a patient with severe abdominal pain includes
  a. administering 100% oxygen.
  b. auscultating for bowel sounds.
  c. giving the patient sips of water.
  d. placing the patient in a supine position.

_____ **94.** Immediately following a generalized motor seizure, most patients are
  a. apneic.
  b. confused.
  c. hyperactive.
  d. awake and alert.

_____ **95.** As you are providing initial ventilations to a patient with apnea using a bag-valve-mask device, you note minimal rise of the chest. You should next
  a. initiate the mouth-to-mask technique.
  b. increase the volume of the ventilations.
  c. switch to a smaller mask for the BVM device.
  d. ensure that a reservoir is attached to the BVM device.

_____ **96.** As you begin your assessment of an unresponsive man who fell approximately 20′ from a roof, you should first
   a. gently shake the patient to confirm unresponsiveness.
   b. gently tilt the patient's head back to assess for breathing.
   c. assess the rate, depth, and regularity of the patient's breathing.
   d. manually stabilize the patient's head and perform a jaw-thrust maneuver.

_____ **97.** A 56-year-old man has labored, shallow breathing at a rate of 28 breaths/min. He is conscious, but extremely restless. Airway management should consist of
   a. a nasal cannula.
   b. a simple face mask.
   c. a nonrebreathing mask.
   d. positive pressure ventilation.

_____ **98.** Indications that artificial ventilations in an apneic adult are ineffective include
   a. a normal heart rate.
   b. improvement of skin color.
   c. asymmetrical rise of the chest.
   d. ventilations given at 12 breaths/min.

_____ **99.** The AED analyzes your pulseless and apneic patient's cardiac rhythm and advises that a shock is indicated. You should
   a. deliver the shock and resume CPR.
   b. ensure that nobody is touching the patient.
   c. perform CPR for 2 minutes and then deliver the shock.
   d. push the analyze button to confirm that a shock is indicated.

_____ **100.** The most appropriate management of a patient who has sustained widespread full-thickness burns following an explosion should consist of applying
   a. oxygen; dry, sterile dressings; warmth; and providing rapid transport.
   b. oxygen; dry; sterile dressings; burn ointment; and providing rapid transport.
   c. oxygen; moist; sterile dressings; warmth; and providing rapid transport.
   d. oxygen; moist; sterile dressings; burn ointment; and providing rapid transport.

_____ **101.** To ensure delivery of the highest concentration of oxygen to your patient using a nonrebreathing mask, you should
   a. set the flow rate to at least 12 L/min.
   b. securely fasten the mask to the patient's face.
   c. make sure that the reservoir bag is preinflated.
   d. cover the one-way valves on the oxygen mask.

——— **Questions 102 to 105 pertain to the following scenario:**———

You arrive at the scene where a 49-year-old woman is found semiconscious on the floor of her living room. The patient's husband tells you that they were watching TV when this condition suddenly developed. No trauma was involved. The patient moans occasionally and has slight cyanosis to her lips.

_____**102.** After performing a head tilt-chin lift maneuver on this patient, you should next
    a. assess her respirations.
    b. determine the need for oxygen.
    c. insert an oropharyngeal airway.
    d. insert a nasopharyngeal airway.

_____**103.** The patient's respirations are at a rate of 26 breaths/min and shallow. The most appropriate management includes
    a. a nasal cannula set at 1 to 6 L/min.
    b. assisted ventilations with 100% oxygen.
    c. a simple face mask set at 10 to 12 L/min.
    d. A nonrebreathing mask set at 15 L/min.

_____**104.** Shallow respirations will result in
    a. decreased tidal volume.
    b. increased tidal volume.
    c. increased oxygen intake.
    d. increased carbon dioxide removal.

_____**105.** Skin will become cyanotic with
    a. an increase in the amount of venous oxygen.
    b. an increase in the amount of arterial oxygen.
    c. a decrease in the amount of arterial oxygen.
    d. a decrease in circulating red blood cells.

——— **Questions 106 to 110 pertain to the following scenario:**———

You are dispatched to the scene of a motorcycle crash in which two patients were injured. Upon arrival, you find that one patient, a 19-year-old woman, is conscious and alert and is being tended to by a police officer for minor scrapes and cuts. The second patient is a 20-year-old man who is found facedown approximately 25' from the motorcycle. He states that he cannot feel or move his legs. Neither patient was wearing a helmet.

_____**106.** After taking body substance isolation precautions, you begin your initial assessment of the man. Your first action should be to
    a. apply an extrication collar.
    b. stabilize his head manually.
    c. evaluate the patency of his airway.
    d. roll him to a supine position.

_____**107.** You have given high concentration oxygen to the man and completed the remainder of your initial assessment. What should you do next?
    a. Obtain baseline vital signs.
    b. Perform a rapid trauma assessment.
    c. Conduct a detailed physical examination.
    d. Immobilize the patient with a vest-style device.

_____**108.** As you are loading the man into the ambulance, the police officer advises you that the woman is refusing EMS treatment and transport. You should next
   a. ask the police officer to obtain a signed refusal from the patient as you proceed to the hospital.
   b. ask the police officer to administer a breathalyzer test to determine if the patient has been drinking alcohol.
   c. advise the patient that she should be transported to the hospital because of the seriousness of the crash.
   d. obtain a signed refusal from the patient and ask the police officer to transport her to the hospital.

_____**109.** While en route to the hospital with the male patient, you begin a detailed physical exam. During the exam, you note that the patient's respiratory rate has increased. You should
   a. immediately notify the receiving facility.
   b. count the number of respirations per minute.
   c. assess his oxygen saturation with a pulse oximeter.
   d. repeat the initial assessment and treat as needed.

_____ **110.** The most reliable indicator of injury to the spinal vertebrae is
   a. lack of pain at the site of the injury.
   b. palpable pain at the site of the injury.
   c. decreased movement on one side of the body.
   d. decreased grip strength in the upper extremities.

_____ **111.** You receive a call for a 3-year-old girl with respiratory distress. When you enter her residence, you see the mother holding the little girl, who does not acknowledge your presence. This finding indicates that the child
   a. has hypoxia.
   b. probably is sleeping.
   c. is afraid of your presence.
   d. is reacting normally for her age.

_____ **112.** Following an apparent febrile seizure, a 4-year-old boy is alert and crying. His skin is warm and moist. The most appropriate management of this child includes
   a. rapidly cooling the child in cold water.
   b. allowing the parents to transport the child.
   c. offering oxygen and providing transport.
   d. keeping the child warm and providing transport.

_____ **113.** You should suspect potential abuse of a 4-year-old child when you encounter
   a. bruises to the anterior tibial area.
   b. curious siblings who are watching you.
   c. purple and yellow bruises to the thighs.
   d. clinging to the parent during your assessment.

_____ **114.** A 30-year-old woman has severe lower abdominal pain and light vaginal bleeding. She tells you that her last menstrual period was 2 months ago. On the basis of these findings, you should suspect
    a. a normal pregnancy.
    b. an ectopic pregnancy.
    c. a spontaneous abortion.
    d. a ruptured ovarian cyst.

_____ **115.** Management of an 18-year-old woman with severe vaginal bleeding includes all of the following, EXCEPT
    a. high concentrations of oxygen.
    b. elevation of the lower extremities.
    c. placing sterile dressings into the vagina.
    d. covering the vagina with a trauma dressing.

_____ **116.** A sudden onset of respiratory distress in a 5-year-old child with no fever most likely is the result of
    a. infection of the lower airways.
    b. inflammation of the upper airway.
    c. a progressive upper airway infection.
    d. obstruction of the airway by a foreign body.

_____ **117.** The most important initial steps of assessing and managing a newborn include
    a. suctioning the airway and obtaining a heart rate.
    b. clearing the airway and keeping the infant warm.
    c. keeping the infant warm and counting respirations.
    d. drying and warming the infant and obtaining an APGAR score.

_____ **118.** Which position is most appropriate for a mother in labor with a prolapsed umbilical cord?
    a. Left lateral recumbent
    b. Left side with legs elevated
    c. Supine with hips elevated
    d. Supine with legs elevated

_____ **119.** When is it most appropriate to clamp and cut the umbilical cord?
    a. As soon as the cord stops pulsating
    b. After the placenta has completely delivered
    c. Before the newborn has taken its first breath
    d. Immediately following delivery of the newborn

_____ **120.** Which of the following statements best describes a mass-casualty incident?
    a. More than five patients are involved.
    b. At least half of the patients are critically injured.
    c. The number of patients overwhelms your resources.
    d. More than three vehicles are involved in the incident.

_____ **121.** In addition to ensuring your own safety, your primary responsibility when functioning at the scene of a violent crime is to
    a. preserve any potential evidence.
    b. appropriately manage the patient.
    c. notify medical control prior to initiating care.
    d. obtain police permission before providing patient care.

_____ **122.** The initial treatment of choice for ventricular fibrillation of short duration, such as a witnessed cardiac arrest is
    a. 100% oxygen delivery.
    b. prompt defibrillation.
    c. CPR for 2 minutes.
    d. cardiac drug therapy.

_____ **123.** While managing a patient in cardiac arrest, you turn the AED on and attach the pads to the patient. When you push the analyze button, the machine signals "low battery" and then ceases to function. The patient subsequently dies. Which of the following statements regarding this case is most correct?
    a. You and your partner may be held liable for negligence.
    b. The crew that preceded you may be held liable for negligence.
    c. The manufacturer of the AED may be held liable for negligence.
    d. Most errors associated with the AED involve equipment failure.

_____ **124.** Following delivery of a newborn, you note that the mother has a moderate amount of vaginal bleeding. The mother is conscious and alert and her vital signs are stable. The most appropriate management of the mother includes
    a. massaging the uterus if signs of shock develop.
    b. administering oxygen and massaging the uterus.
    c. placing a sanitary pad in the vagina and administering oxygen.
    d. treating her for shock and providing immediate transport.

_____ **125.** You are responding to a call for a 2-year-old child who fell from a second-story window. With the mechanism of injury and the age of the patient in mind, you should suspect that the primary injury occurred to the child's
    a. head.
    b. chest.
    c. abdomen.
    d. lower extremities.

_____ **126.** At the peak of the inspiratory phase, the alveoli in the lungs contain
    a. high quantities of carbon dioxide.
    b. minimal levels of oxygen and carbon dioxide.
    c. equal levels of oxygen and carbon dioxide.
    d. more oxygen than carbon dioxide.

_____ **127.** Pulmonary surfactant serves which of the following functions?
   a. It carries fresh oxygen from the lungs to the left side of the heart.
   b. It dilates the bronchioles in the lungs and enhances the flow of air.
   c. It lubricates the alveolar walls and allows them to expand and recoil.
   d. It facilitates the transport of oxygen-poor blood from the right ventricle to the lungs.

———— **Questions 128 to 130 pertain to the following scenario:**————
You receive a call to a restaurant where a 34-year-old man is experiencing shortness of breath. When you arrive, you immediately note that the man has urticaria on his face and arms. He is in obvious respiratory distress, but is awake and alert.

_____ **128.** Suspecting an allergic reaction, your first action should be to
   a. ask the patient if he has an epinephrine auto-injector.
   b. remove the patient's shirt to inspect his chest for urticaria.
   c. obtain a set of baseline vital signs and a SAMPLE history.
   d. place a nonrebreathing mask set at 15 L/min on the patient.

_____ **129.** Epinephrine possesses which of the following effects when it is used to treat anaphylaxis?
   a. As a vasodilator, it increases the blood pressure.
   b. As a vasoconstrictor, it lowers the blood pressure.
   c. As a bronchodilator, it facilitates adequate breathing.
   d. As a bronchoconstrictor, it inhibits the release of chemicals that cause the reaction.

_____ **130.** The patient tells you that he does not have his own epinephrine; however, his wife is allergic to bees and has a prescribed epinephrine auto-injector. You should next
   a. provide transport and consider an ALS rendezvous.
   b. assist the patient with the wife's prescribed epinephrine.
   c. obtain consent from medical control to give the wife's epinephrine to the patient.
   d. assist the patient with one half the usual dose of the wife's epinephrine.

_____ **131.** An elderly man is found unconscious in his kitchen. The patient's wife tells you that her husband has diabetes and that he took his insulin, but did not eat anything. You should suspect
   a. ketoacidosis.
   b. diabetic coma.
   c. hypoglycemia.
   d. hyperglycemia.

_____ **132.** Which of the following statements regarding the function of insulin is most correct?
   a. It stimulates the liver to produce glycogen.
   b. It promotes the entry of glucose from the cell into the bloodstream.
   c. It facilitates the uptake of glucose from the bloodstream into the cell.
   d. It causes the pancreas to produce glucose based on the body's demand.

_____**133.** Which of the following natures of illness is most consistent with a patient with low blood glucose level who is acting bizarre and breathing shallowly?
a. Cardiac compromise
b. Altered mental status
c. Behavioral emergency
d. Respiratory emergency

_____**134.** A 42-year-old man was ejected from his car after it struck a bridge pillar at a high rate of speed. You find him lying approximately 50′ from the car. After manually stabilizing his head, your next action should be to
a. assess the quality of his breathing.
b. grasp the angles of the jaw and lift.
c. administer high-concentration oxygen.
d. determine the patient's level of consciousness.

_____**135.** Which of the following actions is most important when immobilizing a patient with a suspected spinal injury?
a. Immobilize the patient using a vest-style device.
b. Secure the patient's head prior to immobilizing the torso.
c. Select and apply the appropriate size of extrication collar.
d. Assess for range of motion by asking the patient to move the head.

_____**136.** During a soccer game, an 18-year-old woman injured her knee. You note that the knee is in the flexed position and is obviously deformed. Your first action should be to
a. assess her distal circulation.
b. straighten the knee to facilitate immobilization.
c. manually stabilize the leg above and below the knee.
d. immobilize the knee in the position in which it was found.

_____**137.** You have applied a pressure bandage and additional dressings to a large laceration with severe arterial bleeding. The bandages are quickly blood-soaked. You should next
a. elevate the extremity and apply a proximal arterial tourniquet.
b. apply pressure to the pulse point that is most distal to the injury.
c. place additional dressings on the wound until the bleeding stops.
d. remove the bandages and apply pressure at the site of the bleeding.

_____**138.** Which of the following assessment findings would LEAST suggest cardiac compromise?
a. Tachycardia
b. An irregular pulse
c. Palpable pain to the chest
d. Nausea and epigastric pain

_____**139.** Management of an unconscious, breathing patient with a significant cardiac history would include all of the following, EXCEPT
a. analyzing the rhythm with an AED.
b. providing ventilatory support as needed.
c. requesting the presence of an ALS ambulance.
d. obtaining a SAMPLE history from the patient's spouse.

_____**140.** The wall that separates the left and right sides of the heart is the
   a. carina.
   b. septum.
   c. pericardium.
   d. mediastinum.

_____**141.** Prior to administering nitroglycerin to a patient with chest pain, you must
   a. complete a detailed physical examination of the patient.
   b. contact medical control and obtain proper authorization.
   c. make sure that the systolic blood pressure is at least 120 mm Hg.
   d. make sure that the nitroglycerin is prescribed to the patient or a family member.

_____**142.** After the delivery of the first defibrillation with the AED, the patient has a return of a pulse. You should next
   a. provide rapid transport to the hospital.
   b. reanalyze the rhythm for confirmation.
   c. assess the airway and ventilatory status.
   d. remove the AED and apply 100% oxygen.

_____**143.** Which of the following actions would most likely cause a sudden drop in a patient's blood glucose level?
   a. Mild exertion after eating a meal
   b. Eating a meal after taking insulin
   c. Taking too much prescribed insulin
   d. Forgetting to take prescribed insulin

_____**144.** Prior to your arrival at the scene, a near-drowning victim was removed from the water. You should manage the patient's airway appropriately while considering the possibility of
   a. spinal injury.
   b. hyperthermia.
   c. internal bleeding.
   d. airway obstruction.

_____**145.** A soft-tissue injury that results in a flap of torn skin is referred to as
   a. an incision.
   b. an avulsion.
   c. an abrasion.
   d. a laceration.

_____**146.** Following blunt injury to the anterior trunk, a patient is coughing up bright red blood. You should be most suspicious of
   a. intra-abdominal bleeding.
   b. gastrointestinal bleeding.
   c. bleeding within the lungs.
   d. severe myocardial damage.

_____**147.** The effectiveness of chest compressions are most effectively assessed by
    a. listening for a heartbeat with each compression.
    b. carefully measuring the depth of each compression.
    c. palpating for a carotid pulse with each compression.
    d. measuring the systolic blood pressure during compressions.

_____**148.** The position of comfort for a patient with nontraumatic chest pain most commonly is
    a. semisitting.
    b. lateral recumbent.
    c. on the side with the head elevated.
    d. supine with the legs elevated slightly.

_____**149.** Which of the following structures is the primary pacemaker, which sets the normal rate for the heart?
    a. Bundle of His
    b. Purkinje fibers
    c. Sinoatrial node
    d. Atrioventricular node

_____**150.** The middle, muscular layer of the heart is called the
    a. epicardium.
    b. pericardium.
    c. myocardium.
    d. endocardium.

Table 2-1

Practice Final Examination Blueprint

Subtest and # of Items	Questions In Subtest	Minimum Suggested Correct
Airway and Breathing (30)	1,8,9,11,15,23,31,32,56-60, 63,72-74,83,86,95-98, 101-105,126,127	21
Cardiology (25)	13,21,22,24,26,38,41-43, 47,52,80,81,85,87,99,122, 138-142,147-150	18
Trauma (25)	2-4,16,17,19,25,51,53-55, 82,84,100,106,107,109,110, 134-137,144-146	18
Medical (25)	5,14,18,27-29,40,49,50,61, 62,64,89-94,128-133,143	18
Obstetrics and Pediatrics (25)	7,20,34,37,44,45,48,65-71, 111-119,124,125	18
Operations (20)	6,10,12,30,33,35,36,39,46, 75-79,88,108,120,121,123	14
150 ITEMS		**107**

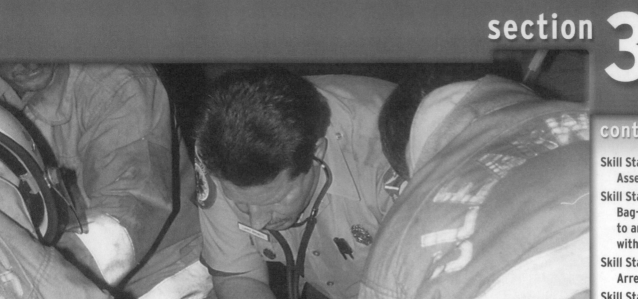

The EMT-Basic Practical Examination

An EMT-Basic candidate is eligible to take the national EMT-B written examination following completion of a state-approved practical examination. Some states use their own skill measurement tools and examination process; however, in many states, the national practical examination process is used to fulfill this requirement.

The skills that comprise the national EMT-Basic practical examination are as follows

1. **Patient Assessment/Management–Trauma**

2. **Patient Assessment/Management–Medical**

3. **Applying a Bag-Valve-Mask Device to an Apneic Patient with a Pulse**

4. **Cardiac Arrest Management/AED**

5. **Spinal Immobilization**
   - Spinal Immobilization–seated, or
   - Spinal Immobilization–supine

6. **Random Basic Skills** (**one** of the following at random)
   - Oxygen administration
   - Airway adjuncts and suctioning
   - Mouth-to-mask ventilation with supplemental oxygen
   - Traction splint
   - Immobilization of a joint injury
   - Immobilization of a long bone fracture
   - Bleeding control and shock management

Notice: The National Registry of EMTs has granted the author the right to reproduce the skill performance checklists contained within this manual, in whole or in part. The National Registry of EMTs is not responsible for the enhancements made to the skill checklists in this publication, nor do they endorse such enhancements.

Skill Station Examiners

The skill station examiners have been chosen based on their expertise in the skill in which they will be evaluating. They will serve as objective recorders of your actions and will provide you with all information necessary to perform the skill. Keep in mind that some skill examiners document more than others. The amount of documentation does not indicate your level of performance in the skill station. Remain focused on what you are doing, not what the examiner is writing or not writing. Upon completion of a skill, the examiner is not allowed to give you feedback or in any way indicate your degree of performance. The skill examiner is unaware of the minimum point values that must be met for each skill. This further ensures maximum objectivity in recording your performance.

The Performance Checklists

The performance checklists for each of the EMT-Basic skills represent a logical fashion in which to perform the skill. Many candidates focus on literally memorizing the sequence of the skill instead of concentrating on and understanding the events that must occur within that sequence.

   When preparing for the practical examination, it is clearly smart to be thoroughly familiar with the performance checklist; however, a healthy understanding of the concept of the skill is far more vital. Just because you miss a few steps in a particular skill does not equate to automatic failure. The reason why candidates do not successfully complete a skill is because they perform actions or fail to perform actions that would result in harm to the patient or themselves. These actions or inactions are what comprise the established critical criteria for each skill.

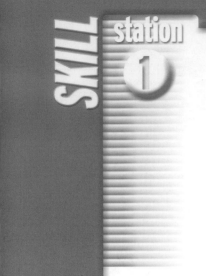

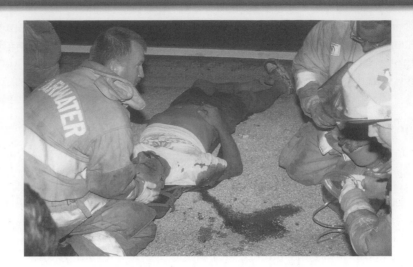

Patient Assessment/Management

The patient assessment and management station for the EMT-B consists of both a trauma and a medical component.

Both the trauma and medical assessment stations require much forethought and verbalization. Your "verbal" treatment should be identical to treatment that you would actually provide to a patient in the field. If you can thoroughly verbalize all aspects of care for the trauma and medical patient, in all likelihood, you will be able to perform safely and effectively in the field.

Skill 1A: Trauma Patient Assessment

Station Time Limit: 10 minutes

Skill Station Objective: This station is designed to test your ability to perform an assessment of a patient with trauma to multiple systems and "voice" treat all conditions and injuries that you discover. You must conduct your assessment as you would in the field to include communicating with your patient. As you conduct your assessment, you must state exactly what you are assessing. Clinical information not obtainable by physical or visual inspection will be given to you after you demonstrate how you would normally obtain that information.

Your Partner(s): You may assume that two EMTs are working with you and they are correctly carrying out the verbal treatments that you indicate.

Skill Examiner Function(s): The skill station examiner will track your time during this station and provide specific clinical information not obtainable by visual or physical inspection. For example, the skill station examiner will provide you with the patient's vital signs, but only if you ask for them. At times, the examiner may ask you for additional information if clarification is needed. For example, if you state that you are placing the patient on "high-flow oxygen," the examiner would ask you how you would accomplish that.

Table 3-1

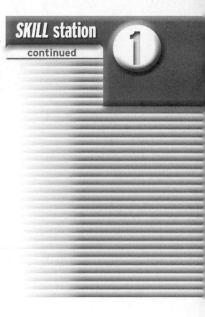

SKILL station
continued
1

Trauma Patient Assessment Performance Checklist

Trauma Patient Assessment			
Takes or verbalizes body substance isolation precautions		1	
SCENE SIZE-UP			
Determines that the scene is safe		1	
Determines the mechanism of injury		1	
Determines the number of patients		1	
Requests additional help if necessary		1	
Considers stabilization of spine		1	
INITIAL ASSESSMENT			
Verbalizes general impression of patient		1	
Determines chief complaint/apparent life threats		1	
Determines responsiveness		1	
Assesses airway and breathing	Performs assessment	1	
	Initiates appropriate oxygen therapy	1	
	Ensures adequate ventilation	1	
	Provides injury management	1	
Assesses circulation	Assesses for and controls major bleeding	1	
	Assesses pulse	1	
	Assesses skin (color, temperature, and condition)	1	
Identifies priority patients and makes transport decision		1	
FOCUSED PHYSICAL EXAM AND HISTORY/RAPID TRAUMA ASSESSMENT			
Selects appropriate assessment (focused or rapid assessment)		1	
Obtains baseline vital signs		1	
Obtains SAMPLE history		1	
DETAILED PHYSICAL EXAMINATION			
Assesses the head	Inspects and palpates the scalp and ears	1	
	Assesses the eyes	1	
	Assesses the facial area, including oral and nasal area	1	
Assesses the neck	Inspects and palpates the neck	1	
	Assesses for jugular venous distention	1	
	Assesses for tracheal deviation	1	
Assesses the chest	Inspects	1	
	Palpates	1	
	Auscultates the chest	1	
Assesses the abdomen/pelvis	Assesses the abdomen	1	
	Assesses the pelvis	1	
	Verbalizes assessment of genitalia/perineum as needed	1	
Assesses the extremities	1 point for each extremity	4	
	Assessment includes inspection, palpation, and assessment of pulses and sensory and motor activities		
Assesses the posterior	Assesses thorax	1	
	Assesses lumbar	1	
Manages secondary injuries and wounds appropriately			
1 point for appropriate management of each injury/wound up to a maximum of 2 points		2	
Verbalizes reassessment of the vital signs		1	
MODELED FROM THE NREMT PERFORMANCE SKILL SHEET		**41**	

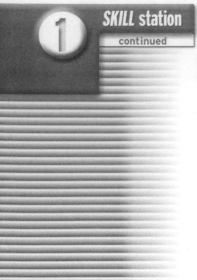

To best prepare for this skill station, you should review the patient assessment and trauma sections of your EMT-Basic textbook. Additionally, you should practice frequently while following the steps of the performance checklist (Table 3-1). If you have recently taken courses such as Basic Trauma Life Support (BTLS) or Prehospital Trauma Life Support (PHTLS), you should be well prepared for this station.

Remember that this is not an evaluation only of your ability to assess a trauma patient. You must integrate the appropriate management within your assessment as well.

Most errors at this station occur because the candidate focuses more on the assessment and less on providing the appropriate management at the appropriate time. Just as you would do on a real call, you must provide immediate care for all life-threatening injuries such as inadequate breathing, altered mental status, and severe bleeding as soon as you discover them.

Critical Criteria: Trauma Patient Assessment/Management

1.   Failure to take or verbalize body substance isolation precautions (BSI).

- So that you do not forget this critical criterion, you might consider physically entering the station with gloves on. The examiner will see this and note that you have taken the appropriate BSI precautions.

2.   Failure to determine scene safety before approaching the patient.

- Just as your chances of serious injury or death would increase dramatically if you do not determine the safety of the scene, so will your chances of not successfully completing this skill if you do not ask whether the scene is safe before making contact with the patient.
- If the examiner tells you that the scene is not safe, you must state what actions you would normally take to ensure its safety (ie, notifying the police, power company, fire department, etc).

3.   Failure to assess for spinal protection.

- This is a determination that you must make after noting the mechanism of injury. Spinal precautions must be taken with all critical trauma patients.
- You can fulfill this critical criterion by simply stating that you will direct your partner to maintain manual stabilization of the head.

4.   Failure to provide spinal protection when indicated.

- Remember, this is a "voice"-treated station. You must verbalize all management that you render. Many candidates fail to verbalize that they had applied an extrication collar or immobilized the patient to a long spine board. (Tip: The best time to apply the extrication collar is immediately after you assess the back of the neck in the rapid trauma assessment.)
- To avoid making this critical error, be sure that you tell the examiner that the patient is fully immobilized prior to loading the patient into the ambulance for transport.

5.   Failure to provide a high concentration of oxygen.

- Remember that ALL critical trauma patients must receive oxygen. Oxygen can be given in one of two forms, either via a nonrebreathing mask set at 15 L/min or via a bag-valve-mask device at 15 L/min during artificial ventilations.
- The appropriate oxygen therapy must be provided to the patient during the initial assessment, immediately after you assess the adequacy of the respirations.

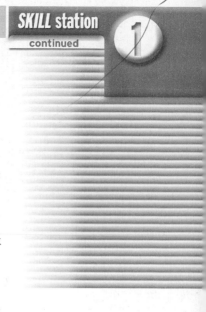

SKILL station
continued
①

6. **Failure to find or manage problems associated with the airway, breathing, hemorrhage, or shock [hypoperfusion].**

    - This is a broad critical criterion that encompasses many areas of assessment and management. The following is a breakdown of each area with suggestions for ensuring that all of these major areas are covered:
      - Airway
        - Open the airway using the appropriate technique (the jaw-thrust maneuver) and at the appropriate time, which is when you direct your partner to manually stabilize the head.
        - Be sure to provide suction if any secretions such as blood or vomitus are in the airway. You must clear the airway before you can assess and manage it.
      - Breathing
        - Deliver the appropriate oxygenation or ventilation to the patient. If the patient is breathing adequately, at a minimum, 100% oxygen via a nonrebreathing mask must be provided. If the patient is breathing inadequately with shallow or irregular respirations or has apnea, you must provide artificial ventilations with 100% supplemental oxygen and reservoir attached.
        - Locate and manage any problems such as a sucking chest wound, flail chest, etc that could impair the airway and breathing.
      - Hemorrhage
        - When you assess circulation during the initial assessment, you must inquire about severe bleeding. If it is present, you must address it immediately. Remember, you can ask one of your EMT partners to take care of managing it for you.
        - To provide you with information about the possibility of severe bleeding, listen carefully to what the examiner tells you when you inquire about the general impression (ie, "the patient is found unconscious in a large pool of blood").
        - ALL severe bleeding must be stopped immediately when discovered, but you must assess for it in order to find it.
      - Shock [Hypoperfusion]
        - Be sure to recognize the signs and symptoms of shock and initiate management early. If the patient has cool, clammy skin, tachycardia, and is restless during the initial assessment, begin managing the patient for shock at once (ie, place a blanket over the patient, elevate the legs, and apply oxygen) and continue with this treatment throughout the scenario.

7. **Failure to differentiate the patient's need for transport from the need for continued assessment at the scene.**

    - If you discover any abnormal findings in the initial assessment, such as a significant mechanism of injury, problems with airway, breathing, or circulation, or an altered mental status, you must perform a rapid trauma assessment.
      - Tip: You only perform rapid trauma assessments on critically injured patients. If a rapid trauma assessment is indicated, the patient is considered to be a "load and go." As soon as the rapid trauma assessment is completed, make sure the patient is fully immobilized and state that you are transporting the patient. Baseline vital signs and SAMPLE history can be obtained en route.
    - A detailed physical examination should be performed en route to the hospital when managing a critically injured patient. If you forget to say out loud that you are en route to the hospital (even if you meant to say it) and you begin a detailed exam at the scene, the examiner will assume that you have not transported the patient yet. Remember: verbalize, verbalize, and verbalize!

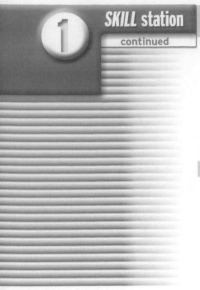

SKILL station *continued*

8. **Failure to assess the airway, breathing, and circulation before performing a detailed physical examination.**

- An initial assessment is performed on ALL patients, regardless of their degree of injury. Following the initial assessment, you will progress in one of two directions:
  - Critical patient = rapid trauma assessment
  - Noncritical patient = focused physical examination
- You must assess for and manage all problems with the ABCs before performing any further assessment of the patient. With the exception of the scene size-up, NOTHING precedes the initial assessment.

9. **Failure to transport patient within the 10-minute time limit.**

- Do not get this confused with "did not complete the station within the 10-minute time limit."
- There is an overall time limit of 10 minutes to complete this station; however, the critical component is that the patient must be transported prior to expiration of this time limit.
  - Tip: Even if you transport the patient with 2 minutes left in the station, you still must conduct your detailed physical examination, each component of which is worth a point. If you do not accrue enough total points, you could still fail. Be swift, but cover all of your bases.

Skill 1B: Medical Patient Assessment

Station Time Limit: 10 minutes.

Skill Station Objective: This station is designed to test your ability to perform an assessment of a patient with a chief complaint of a medical nature and "voice" treat all conditions that you discover. You must conduct your assessment as you would in the field to include communicating with your patient. As you conduct your assessment, you must state everything you are assessing. Clinical information not obtainable by physical or visual inspection will be given to you after you demonstrate how you would normally gain that information.

Your Partner(s): You may assume that two EMTs are working with you and they are correctly carrying out the verbal treatments that you indicate.

Skill Examiner Function(s): The skill station examiner will track your time during this station and provide specific clinical information not obtainable by visual or physical inspection. For example, the skill station examiner will provide you with the patient's vital signs, but only if you ask for them. At times, the examiner may ask you for additional information if clarification is needed. For example, if you state that you are placing the patient on "high-flow oxygen," the examiner would ask you how you would accomplish that.

Table 3-2

SKILL station continued **1**

Medical Patient Assessment Performance Checklist

Medical Patient Assessment		
Takes or verbalizes body substance isolation precautions	1	
SCENE SIZE-UP		
Determines the scene is safe	1	
Determines the mechanism of injury	1	
Determines the number of patients	1	
Requests additional help if necessary	1	
Considers stabilization of spine	1	
INITIAL ASSESSMENT		
Verbalizes general impression of the patient	1	
Determines chief complaint/apparent life threats	1	
Determines responsiveness and level of consciousness	1	
Assesses airway and breathing — Performs assessment	1	
Initiates appropriate oxygen therapy	1	
Ensures adequate ventilation	1	
Assesses circulation — Assesses for and controls major bleeding	1	
Assesses pulse	1	
Assesses skin (color, temperature, and condition)	1	
Identifies priority patients and makes transport decision	1	
FOCUSED PHYSICAL EXAM AND HISTORY/RAPID ASSESSMENT		
Signs and Symptoms (Assess history of present illness)	1	

Respiratory	**Cardiac**	**Altered Mental Status**	**Allergic Reaction**
*Onset?	*Onset?	*Description of the episode	*History of allergies?
*Provoking factors?	*Provoking factors?	*Onset?	*What were you exposed to?
*Quality?	*Quality?	*Duration?	^How were you exposed?
*Radiation?	*Radiation?	*Associated symptoms?	*Effects?
*Severity?	*Severity?	*Evidence of trauma?	*Progressions?
*Time?	*Time?	*Interventions?	*Interventions?
*Interventions?	*Interventions?	*Seizures?	
		*Fever?	

Poisoning/ Overdose	**Environmental Emergency**	**Obstetrics**	**Behavioral**
*Substance?	*Source?	*Are you pregnant?	*How do you feel?
*When did you ingest/become exposed?	*Environment?	*How long have you been pregnant?	*Determine suicidal tendencies
*How much did you ingest?	*Duration?	*Pain or contractions?	*Is the patient a threat to self or others?
*Over what time period?	*Loss of consciousness?	*Bleeding or discharge?	*Is there a medical problem?
*Interventions?	*Effects— General or local?	*Do you feel the need to push?	*Past medical history?
*Estimated weight?		*Last menstrual period?	*Interventions?
*Effects?		*Crowning?	*Medications?

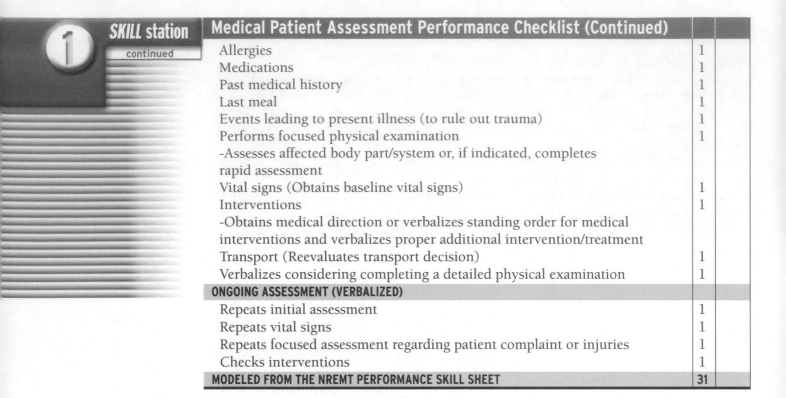

Medical Patient Assessment Performance Checklist (Continued)		
Allergies	1	
Medications	1	
Past medical history	1	
Last meal	1	
Events leading to present illness (to rule out trauma)	1	
Performs focused physical examination	1	
-Assesses affected body part/system or, if indicated, completes rapid assessment		
Vital signs (Obtains baseline vital signs)	1	
Interventions	1	
-Obtains medical direction or verbalizes standing order for medical interventions and verbalizes proper additional intervention/treatment		
Transport (Reevaluates transport decision)	1	
Verbalizes considering completing a detailed physical examination	1	
ONGOING ASSESSMENT (VERBALIZED)		
Repeats initial assessment	1	
Repeats vital signs	1	
Repeats focused assessment regarding patient complaint or injuries	1	
Checks interventions	1	
MODELED FROM THE NREMT PERFORMANCE SKILL SHEET	31	

Reviewing the patient assessment and medical emergencies chapters of an EMT-Basic textbook, as well as frequent practice using the performance checklist (Table 3-2) will prepare you well for this station.

Unlike with trauma patients, management of medical patients can be more complex because you are unable to see what you are treating. You must rely on your assessment skills, specifically the focused history and physical examination, in order to determine what is wrong with the patient so that you can render the most appropriate management.

Lack of success in the medical assessment station typically is secondary to the candidate's inability to form a plausible field impression, which subsequently leads the candidate down the wrong path with regard to the appropriate management. Remember, knowing which questions to ask, based on the patient's chief complaint, will undoubtedly determine whether or not you provide the most appropriate care.

Critical Criteria: Medical Patient Assessment/Management

1.   Failure to take or verbalize BSI precautions.
  • So that you do not forget this critical criterion, you might consider physically entering the station with gloves on. The examiner will see this and note that you have taken the appropriate BSI precautions.

2.   Failure to determine scene safety before approaching the patient.
  • Just as your chances of serious injury or death would increase dramatically if you do not determine the safety of the scene, so will your chances of not successfully completing this skill if you do not ask whether the scene is safe before making contact with the patient.
  • If the examiner tells you that the scene is not safe, you must state what actions you would normally take to ensure its safety (ie, notifying the police, power company, fire department, etc).

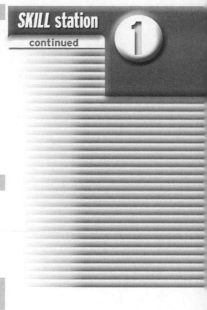

SKILL station

continued

1

3. **Failure to obtain medical direction or verbalize standing orders for medical interventions.**
   - Remember, you *must* contact medical control and obtain authorization to perform the following:
     - Assist with an epinephrine auto-injector, prescribed inhaler, or nitroglycerin.
     - Administer activated charcoal or oral glucose.
   - If the patient does not require any interventions other than those mentioned above, you must still verbalize that by standing orders, you would administer oxygen or assist ventilations, whichever is most appropriate for the situation. In cases where oxygen is the only therapy needed, you would not be required to contact medical control.

4. **Failure to provide a high concentration of oxygen.**
   - Remember that this station requires that 100% oxygen be given. Oxygen can be given in one of two forms, either via a nonrebreathing mask set at 15 L/min or via a bag-valve-mask device at 15 L/min during artificial ventilations.
   - The appropriate oxygen therapy must be provided to the patient during the initial assessment, immediately after you assess the adequacy of the respirations.

5. **Failure to find or manage problems associated with the airway, breathing, hemorrhage, or shock [hypoperfusion].**
   - This is a broad critical criterion that encompasses many areas of assessment and management. The following is a breakdown of each area with suggestions for ensuring that all of these major areas are covered:
     - Airway
       - Open the airway using the appropriate technique. If you are unsure about the possibility of trauma and the patient has an altered mental status, use the jaw-thrust maneuver. Otherwise, use the head tilt-chin lift maneuver.
       - Be sure to provide suction if any secretions (such as blood or vomitus) are in the airway. You must clear the airway before you can assess and manage it.
     - Breathing
       - Deliver the appropriate oxygenation or ventilation to the patient. If the patient is breathing adequately, at a minimum, 100% oxygen via a nonrebreathing mask must be provided. If the patient is breathing inadequately (with shallow or irregular respirations or apnea), you must provide artificial ventilations with 100% supplemental oxygen and reservoir attached.
     - Hemorrhage
       - When you assess circulation during the initial assessment, you must inquire about severe bleeding. If it is present, you must address it immediately. Remember, you can ask one of your EMT partners to take care of managing it for you.
       - To provide you with information about the possibility of severe bleeding, listen carefully to what the examiner tells you when you inquire about the general impression (ie, "the patient is found unconscious in a large pool of blood").
       - ALL severe bleeding must be stopped immediately when discovered, but you must assess for it in order to find it.
       - You must not assume the patient is not bleeding just because this is a medical assessment station.
     - Shock [Hypoperfusion]
       - Be sure to recognize the signs and symptoms of shock and initiate management early. If the patient has cool, clammy skin, tachycardia, and is restless during the initial assessment, begin managing the patient for shock at once (ie, place a blanket over the patient, elevate the legs, apply oxygen) and continue with this treatment throughout the scenario.

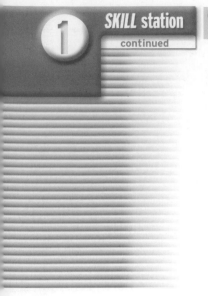

SKILL station
continued

6. **Failure to differentiate the patient's need for transport from the need for continued assessment at the scene.**

- Any patient with airway, breathing, or circulation problems will require immediate transport. General guidelines regarding your actions after the initial assessment, based on the type of patient, follow:
  - Unresponsive patient: Rapid assessment (same technique as the rapid trauma assessment), baseline vital signs and SAMPLE history, interventions, immediate transport, detailed physical examination en route to the hospital.
    - Remember, you will have to provide interventions such as airway and breathing support throughout this sequence of events.
  - Responsive patient, but with ABC problems: Focused history and physical examination, baseline vital signs and SAMPLE history, interventions, immediate transport.
    - Remember, you will have to provide interventions such as airway and breathing support throughout this sequence of events.
- Only unresponsive patients receive a detailed physical examination, which is conducted en route to the hospital. Your only actions at the scene should be the initial assessment and either a rapid assessment or focused history and physical examination.

7. **Failure to assess the airway, breathing, and circulation before performing a detailed or focused history/physical examination.**

- An initial assessment is performed on ALL patients, regardless of their degree of illness. Following the initial assessment, you will progress in one of two directions:
  - Unresponsive patient = rapid assessment
  - Responsive patient = focused physical examination
- You must assess for and manage all problems with the ABCs before performing any further assessment of the patient. With the exception of the scene size-up, NOTHING precedes the initial assessment.

8. **Failure to ask questions about the present illness.**

- Based on the patient's chief complaint, you must ask questions that are pertinent to that complaint (history of present illness). This will provide you with the information that you need in order to render the most appropriate care. For example, you should ask the following questions of a patient with a complaint of a cardiac nature:
  - Onset: was it sudden or progressive?
  - Provocation/Palliation: does anything make the pain worse or better?
  - Quality: describe the pain (sharp, dull, crushing, etc).
  - Radiation: does the pain stay in one place or does it move around?
  - Severity: on a scale of 1 to 10, with 1 being no pain and 10 being the worst pain you have ever felt, how would you rate the pain you are feeling right now?
  - Time: when did the pain begin?
  - Interventions: did you take any medications (ie, prescribed nitroglycerin) prior to EMS arrival?
- In order to receive a point for this critical criterion, you must ask a certain number of questions, based on the chief complaint. Remember to ask all of the pertinent questions for each type of patient. Do not memorize a certain number of them just to get the point. Here are the *minimum* number of questions that must be asked for each type of patient that you may encounter in this station:
  - Respiratory: 5 questions.
  - Cardiac: 5 questions.
  - Altered Mental Status: 6 questions.

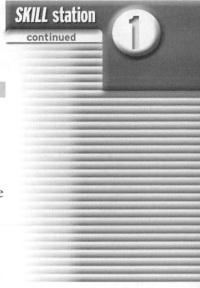

- Allergic reaction: 4 questions.
- Poisoning/Overdose: 5 questions.
- Environmental Emergency: 4 questions.
- Obstetrics: 5 questions.
- Behavioral: 4 questions.

9. Administers a dangerous or inappropriate intervention.

- Following are some clear examples of dangerous or inappropriate interventions:
  - Administers oral glucose or activated charcoal to a patient who is unable to swallow.
  - Assists a patient with nitroglycerin or an inhaler that is not prescribed to *the patient*.
  - Does not allow a patient with breathing difficulty (or any other patient) to assume the most comfortable position.
  - Forces an oropharyngeal airway on a patient who continues to gag.

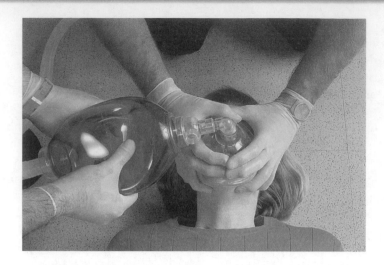

Applying a Bag-Valve-Mask Device to an Apneic Patient with a Pulse

Station Time Limit: 5 minutes

Skill Station Objective: This station is designed to test your ability to ventilate a patient using a bag-valve-mask device. There are no bystanders, and artificial ventilation has not been initiated. The only patient management required is airway management and ventilatory support. You must initially ventilate the patient for 30 seconds. You will be evaluated on the appropriateness of ventilatory volumes. You will then be informed that a second rescuer has arrived, and you will be instructed to control the airway and the mask seal while the second rescuer provides ventilation.

Your Partner(s): A partner will arrive as advised by the examiner and you will resume the two-person bag-valve-mask technique. The EMT assistant will do only what you instruct him or her to do.

Skill Examiner Function(s): The skill station examiner will track your time during this station and observe the effectiveness of your ventilations for at least 30 seconds. The skill station examiner also will advise you when the second rescuer arrives. The examiner may serve as the second rescuer.

SKILL station
continued

Table 3-3

BVM Device–Apneic Patient Performance Checklist

BVM Device-Apneic Patient		
Takes or verbalizes body substance isolation precautions	1	
Verbalizes opening the airway	1	
Verbalizes inserting an airway adjunct	1	
Selects the appropriately sized mask	1	
Creates a proper mask-to-face seal	1	
Ventilates the patient at proper rate with adequate volume (**The examiner must witness this step for at least 30 seconds**)	1	
Connects reservoir and oxygen	1	
Adjusts liter flow to 15 L/min or greater	1	
THE EXAMINER INDICATES ARRIVAL OF A SECOND EMT. THE SECOND EMT IS INSTRUCTED TO VENTILATE THE PATIENT WHILE THE CANDIDATE CONTROLS THE MASK AND THE AIRWAY		
Verbalizes reopening the airway	1	
Creates a proper mask-to-face seal	1	
Instructs assistant to resume ventilations at proper rate with adequate volume (**The examiner must witness this step for at least 30 seconds**)	1	
MODELED FROM THE NREMT PERFORMANCE SKILL SHEET	11	

Critical Criteria: Applying a bag-valve-mask device to an apneic patient with a pulse

1. Failure to take or verbalize BSI precautions.

- So that you do not forget this critical criterion, you might consider physically entering the station with gloves on. The examiner will see this and note that you have taken the appropriate BSI precautions.

2. Failure to immediately ventilate the patient.

- Immediately means immediately. As soon as you are instructed to begin, you must open the patient's airway and immediately initiate artificial ventilations with the bag-valve-mask device.
- Because this station is testing only your ability to perform ventilations using a bag-valve-mask device, not the technique of inserting an airway adjunct, you will verbalize the insertion of an airway adjunct.
- You are required to ventilate the manikin with room air for at least 30 seconds. Do not attempt to connect the reservoir and supplemental oxygen during this time or the examiner likely will mark you off as not "immediately" ventilating the patient.

3. Interrupts ventilations for more than 20 seconds.

- Most candidates have problems in this area when they attach the supplemental oxygen and reservoir.
- Make sure that, prior to beginning this station, you are aware of the location of all of your equipment. The reservoir should be in sight, where you will be able to find it easily.

4. Failure to provide a high concentration of oxygen.

- After initially ventilating the manikin with room air for 30 seconds, you must attach supplemental oxygen tubing and a reservoir. Be sure that you verbalize to the examiner that you have set the oxygen flowmeter to 15 L/min or physically set the flowmeter. This station does not require you to assemble the oxygen tank and regulator.

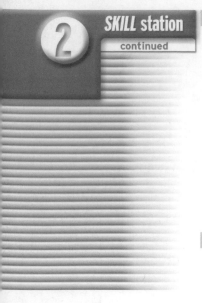

5. Failure to provide or direct the assistant to provide proper volume per breath or rate.

- During the 30 seconds in which the examiner must witness your ventilations, as well as the ventilations provided during the integration of the second rescuer, you are only allowed one inadequate ventilation.
  - A ventilation is considered inadequate if the manikin's chest does not rise or rises minimally.
- The single most common problem encountered when using the bag-valve-mask device is difficulty in maintaining an adequate mask-to-face seal. Failure to maintain the seal will result in inadequate volumes. If you have small hands or if this is easier for you, hold the mask firmly to the manikin's face and squeeze the bag against your leg.
- When your partner is integrated into the station, you should use the "C-clamp" method of securing the mask to the manikin's face.

6. Failure to allow adequate exhalation.

- This can occur if you ventilate the manikin too fast. DO NOT HYPERVENTILATE THE PATIENT.
- Ventilate in the range of 10 to 12 breaths/min and watch for the chest to fall completely before initiating the next ventilation.
- If necessary, count 1–1000, 2–1000, 3–1000, etc, to ensure the appropriate rate of ventilation.

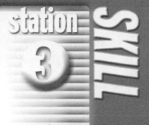

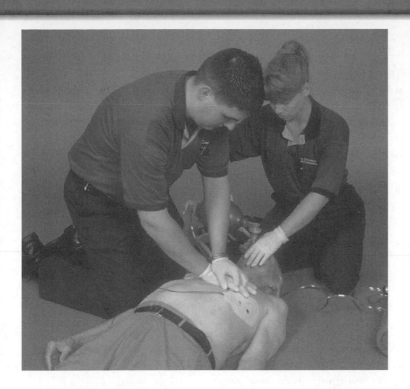

Cardiac Arrest Management/AED

Station Time Limit: 15 minutes

Skill Station Objective: This station is designed to test your ability to manage a prehospital cardiac arrest by integrating CPR skills, defibrillation, airway adjuncts, and patient and scene management skills. As you arrive on the scene, you will encounter a patient in cardiac arrest. A first responder will be present performing one-rescuer CPR. You must immediately establish control of the scene and begin resuscitation of the patient with an automated external defibrillator (AED). At the appropriate time, the patient's airway must be controlled and you must ventilate *or* direct ventilation of the patient using adjunctive equipment.

Your Partner(s): You will have an EMT assistant and a "first responder" in this station. The EMT assistant and first responder will do only what you instruct them to do.

Skill Examiner Function(s): The skill station examiner will track your time during this station and observe your actions as well as those of your partners. The skill station examiner may function as the EMT assistant as needed.

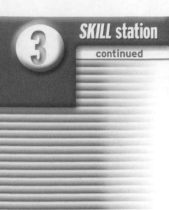

SKILL station
continued

Table 3-4

Cardiac Arrest Management/AED Performance Checklist

Assessment		
Takes or verbalizes body substance isolation precautions	1	
Briefly questions rescuer about arrest events	1	
Turns on AED power	1	
Attaches AED to patient	1	
Directs rescuer to stop CPR and ensures all individuals are clear of the patient	1	
Initiates analysis of the rhythm	1	
Delivers shock	1	
Directs resumption of CPR	1	
TRANSITION		
Gathers additional information about the arrest event	1	
Confirms effectiveness of CPR (ventilations and compressions)	1	
INTEGRATION		
Verbalizes or directs insertion of a simple airway adjunct (oral/nasal airway)	1	
Ventilates or directs ventilation of patient	1	
Assures high concentration of oxygen is delivered to the patient	1	
Assures adequate CPR continues without unnecessary/prolonged interruption	1	
Continues CPR for 2 minutes	1	
Directs rescuer to stop CPR and ensures all individuals are clear of the patient	1	
Initiates analysis of the rhythm	1	
Delivers shock	1	
Directs resumption of CPR	1	
TRANSPORTATION		
Verbalizes transportation of the patient	1	
MODELED FROM THE NREMT PERFORMANCE SKILL SHEET	**20**	

To facilitate your progression through the cardiac arrest station, each of the four components and the actions that should take place within each component will be discussed.

Assessment

- During the assessment phase, after you have taken the appropriate BSI precautions, you must ask the first responder the following questions regarding the events of the cardiac arrest, without interrupting CPR in progress:
  - How long has the patient been in cardiac arrest?
  - How long has CPR been in progress?
- After determining the events of the cardiac arrest, you should turn on the AED and attach the AED pads to the patient; *this should be done without interrupting CPR.*
- After the AED is turned on and connected to the patient, you should initiate analysis of the rhythm. Remember to make sure that all rescuers are clear of the patient during this phase.
- You will deliver *one* shock with the AED. Following are important points to remember during and after delivery of this shock:

SKILL station
continued
3

- Make sure that no rescuers are in contact with the patient prior to delivering the shock.
- Resume CPR *immediately* after delivering the shock.

Transition

- During the transition phase, you should instruct your EMT assistant and the first responder to resume two-rescuer CPR.
- Assess CPR effectiveness by palpating for a carotid or femoral pulse while chest compressions are being performed.
- You should ask any additional questions regarding the cardiac arrest as well as any past medical history and the events leading up to the cardiac arrest at this point.

Integration

- At this point, you must integrate the appropriate airway management into the scenario. *This must be accomplished without interrupting chest compressions.*
- You will verbalize that you would measure and insert an oropharyngeal airway and then ventilate or direct ventilation of the patient using one of the following ventilation devices:
  - Bag-mask device
  - Pocket mask device
- After five cycles (approximately 2 minutes) of CPR, ensure that nobody is in contact with the patient, reanalyze the patient's cardiac rhythm, and deliver *one* shock if indicated. Remember to resume CPR *immediately* after the shock has been delivered.

Transportation

- During this phase, you must verbalize that you would place the patient onto a long spine board, continue CPR, and initiate rapid transport to the hospital.

Critical Criteria: Cardiac Arrest Management/AED

1. Failure to take or verbalize BSI precautions.
- So that you do not forget this critical criterion, you might consider physically entering the station with gloves on. The examiner will see this and note that you have taken the appropriate BSI precautions.

2. Failure to evaluate the need for immediate use of the AED.
- Remember that ventricular fibrillation (V-fib) is the most common initial cardiac dysrhythmia observed during the first few minutes of cardiac arrest in adults.
- Defibrillation is the most important treatment for V-fib.
- Apply the defibrillation pads while chest compressions are being performed; doing so will minimize unnecessary interruptions in CPR.

3. Failure to immediately direct initiation/resumption of CPR at appropriate times.
- There are only two situations in which CPR should not be in progress throughout this station:
  - When you are analyzing the patient's cardiac rhythm.
  - When you are delivering a shock.

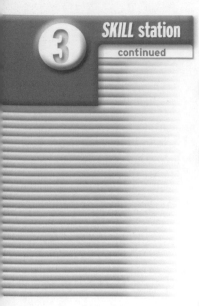

- It is critical to resume CPR *immediately* after any shock. Forgetting to direct the resumption of CPR is not as uncommon as you may think, and it should not be assumed that CPR is in progress or is continuing. Remember, your assistant and the first responder will do *nothing* without your direction.

4. Failure to ensure that all individuals were clear of the patient before delivering a shock.

- I'm clear, you're clear, we're ALL clear.
- Verbally *and* visually make sure that no one is in contact with the patient before delivering any shock.

5. Failure to operate the AED properly or safely (inability to deliver a shock).

- The AED is a very simplistic machine. Following are the steps for properly using the AED to deliver a shock:
- Turn the AED on.
- Apply the pads to the patient's bare chest.
- Ensure that no one is in contact with the patient.
- Push the analyze button (if there is one; many AEDs auto-analyze).
- Recheck to make sure no one is in contact with the patient and deliver one shock if indicated.

6. Prevented the defibrillator from delivering any shock.

- AEDs have a high specificity for recognizing shockable rhythms. If a shock is advised, deliver it without delay. Do not reanalyze to confirm that a shock is indicated.
- Do not remove the AED pads from the patient at any time.
- Do not disconnect the AED cable from the AED at any time.

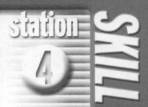

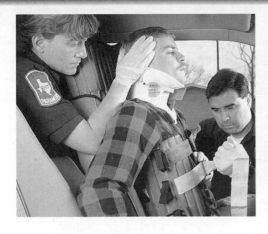 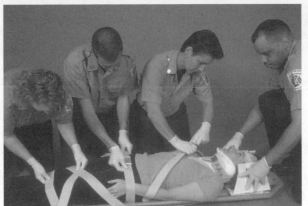

Spinal Immobilization

You will be required to demonstrate immobilization of **either** a seated patient **or** a supine patient. The determination as to which skill you will be tested on is at the discretion of the examination coordinator. Some coordinators use a "draw from the hat" method of determining which skill you will be evaluated on. This ensures fairness and a totally random method of determination.

Skill 4A: Spinal Immobilization (Seated)

Station Time Limit: 10 minutes

Skill Station Objective: This station is designed to test your ability to provide spinal immobilization on a patient using a half-spine immobilization device (either a short spine board or a vest-style device). You and an EMT assistant arrive on the scene of an automobile crash. The scene is safe and there is only one patient. The EMT assistant has completed the initial assessment and no critical conditions requiring intervention were found. For the purpose of this station, the patient's vital signs remain stable. You are required to treat the specific, isolated problem of an unstable spine using a half-spine immobilization device. You are responsible for the direction and subsequent actions of the EMT assistant. Transferring the patient to the long spine board should be accomplished verbally.

Your Partner(s): You will have an EMT assistant in this station. The EMT assistant will do only what you instruct him or her to do.

Skill Examiner Function(s): The skill station examiner will track your time during this station and observe your actions as well as those of your EMT assistant. After completion of the skill, the examiner will check the effectiveness of immobilization by attempting to manipulate the device.

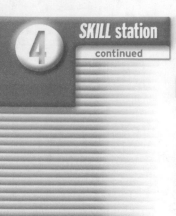

SKILL station
continued

Table 3-5

Spinal Immobilization (Seated) Performance Checklist

Spinal Immobilization (Seated)		
Takes or verbalizes body substance isolation precautions	1	
Directs assistant to place and maintain patient's head in a neutral in-line position	1	
Directs assistant to maintain manual immobilization of the head	1	
Assesses motor, sensory, and distal circulatory function in the extremities	1	
Applies appropriately sized extrication collar	1	
Positions the immobilization device behind the patient	1	
Secures the device to the patient's torso	1	
Evaluates torso fixation and adjusts as necessary	1	
Evaluates and pads behind the patient's head as necessary	1	
Secures the patient's head to the device	1	
Verbalizes moving the patient to a long board	1	
Reassesses motor, sensory, and distal circulatory function in the extremities	1	
MODELED FROM THE NREMT PERFORMANCE SKILL SHEET	**12**	

Critical Criteria: Spinal Immobilization (Seated)

1. Failure to immediately direct or take manual immobilization of the head.
- ANY skill that involves trauma assessment or management begins with your making sure that the patient's head is in a neutral, in-line position. This skill is no different.
- Use your partner, because that is his or her intended purpose.

2. Failure to properly apply an appropriately sized cervical collar before ordering release of the manual immobilization.
- Do not be confused by this statement. Your partner must not release manual stabilization of the patient's head until the patient is *fully* immobilized in the device.
- To ensure the most appropriately sized cervical collar, measure from the top of the patient's shoulder to just below the earlobe. A collar that is not the correct size will cause either flexion or extension of the patient's neck.

3. Releases or orders release of manual immobilization before it was maintained mechanically.
- To best avoid making this mistake, tell your partner to maintain manual stabilization of the patient's head and do not allow him or her to release it until after you have reassessed the patient's distal pulses and neurologic status.
- There is nothing that says your partner must let go of the patient's head after the device is fully applied.
- Remember, the patient is not considered fully immobilized until the entire device is applied.

4. Manipulates or moves the patient excessively, causing potential spinal compromise.
- Ensure that you inform your partner that no patient moves will take place without his or her command.
- All patient moves, regardless of how slight, must be uniform, and the patient must be moved as a unit at the command of the person maintaining stabilization of the patient's head.
- Do not be too rough when applying the immobilization device.

SKILL station
continued
4

5. Immobilizes the head to the device *before* the device was sufficiently secured to the torso.

- Securing the patient's head to the device prior to securing the torso may cause unnecessary movement of the neck when the straps are applied and secured to the torso.
- Do not mechanically immobilize the head until you have *completely* immobilized the torso. Candidates commonly will position the device in its entirety and then go back and tighten the straps. This is a bad practice that should be avoided.

6. Device moves excessively up, down, left, or right on the patient's torso.

- To ensure the most effective immobilization of the torso, when placing the device behind the patient, make sure that the device fits snugly underneath the patient's arms.
- After you have positioned but not secured the torso, step back and look at the patient to make sure that the device is centered, then secure the straps.

7. Head immobilization allows for excessive movement.

- Be sure to use the most appropriately sized cervical collar.
- Many candidates think that the pad for the back of the patient's head must be used simply because it is in the case with the device. In reality, only a small percentage of patients (usually those with "hunchbacks") will require the pad. Most of the time, this pillow device is not needed.
- To ensure effective immobilization of the patient's head, follow this recommended sequence:
  - Position the device behind the patient (snug fit under the arms).
  - When your partner calls for the move, move the patient as a unit until he or she is sitting *completely* back into the device. The spinal cord ends well above the waist; therefore, it is acceptable to flex the patient at the waist to ensure that the patient is seated properly.
  - Remember that the area between the lower back (lumbar) and the back of the patient's head must be in an in-line position at all times.

8. Torso fixation inhibits chest rise, resulting in respiratory compromise.

- To ensure adequate, yet not asphyxiating, security of the torso, ask the patient to take in a deep breath and hold it until you have secured the strap. Repeat this step until all of the torso straps are secured. This will allow for adequate chest expansion within the secured torso.
- Ask the patient if he or she is comfortable. If the patient is not comfortable, you can loosen the torso straps and secure them again as outlined above.

9. Upon completion of immobilization, the head is not in a neutral, in-line position.

- Remember: do not use the posterior padding device simply because it is there. Using the device pushes the head forward. Unnecessary use of this device probably is one of the most common reasons that candidates fail to effectively immobilize the head.
- Be sure to use the appropriately sized cervical collar, as explained earlier.

10. Failure to reassess motor, sensory, and circulatory functions in *each* extremity after verbalizing that immobilization to the long backboard is complete.

- Although you are only required to assess motor, sensory, and circulatory function after you have completed immobilization and stated that the patient has been moved to the long backboard, you should get into the habit of checking these functions three times. You should check them before and after the short device is placed and then after verbalizing that the patient is immobilized to the long backboard. The more you check it, the less chance you have of forgetting.

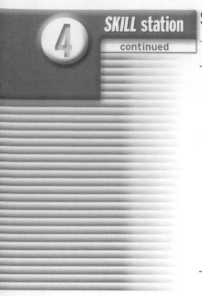

SKILL station
continued

Skill 4B: Spinal Immobilization (Supine)

Station Time Limit: 10 minutes

Skill Station Objective: This station is designed to test your ability to provide spinal immobilization on a patient using a long spine immobilization device. You and an EMT assistant arrive on the scene of an automobile crash. The scene is safe and there is only one patient. The assistant EMT has completed the initial assessment and no critical conditions requiring intervention were found. For the purpose of this station, the patient's vital signs remain stable. You are required to treat the specific, isolated problem of an unstable spine using a long spine immobilization device. You should use the help of the EMT assistant and the evaluator. The EMT assistant should control the patient's head and cervical spine while you and the evaluator move the patient to the immobilization device. You are responsible for the direction and subsequent actions of the EMT assistant.

Your Partner(s): You will have an EMT assistant in this station. The EMT assistant will do only what you instruct him or her to do.

Skill Examiner Function(s): The skill station examiner will track your time during this station and observe your actions as well as those of your EMT assistant. The examiner also will assist you in transferring the patient to the immobilization device.

Table 3-6

Spinal Immobilization (Supine) Performance Checklist

Spinal Immobilization (Supine)		
Takes or verbalizes body substance isolation precautions	1	
Directs assistant to place and maintain patient's head in a neutral in-line position	1	
Directs assistant to maintain manual immobilization of the head	1	
Assesses motor, sensory, and distal circulatory function in the extremities	1	
Applies appropriately sized extrication collar	1	
Positions the immobilization device appropriately	1	
Moves patient onto the device without compromising the integrity of the spine	1	
Applies padding to voids between the torso and the board as necessary	1	
Immobilizes the patient's torso to the device	1	
Evaluates and pads behind the patient's head as necessary	1	
Immobilizes the patient's head to the device	1	
Secures the patient's legs to the device	1	
Secures the patient's arms to the device	1	
Reassesses motor, sensory, and distal circulatory function in the extremities	1	
MODELED FROM THE NREMT PERFORMANCE SKILL SHEET	**14**	

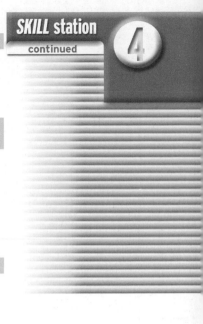

SKILL station
continued
4

Critical Criteria: Spinal Immobilization (Supine)

1. Failure to immediately direct or take manual immobilization of the head.

- ANY skill that involves trauma assessment or management begins with your making sure that the patient's head is in a neutral, in-line position. This skill is no different.
- Use your partner, because that is his or her intended purpose.

2. Failure to properly apply an appropriately sized cervical collar before ordering release of the manual immobilization.

- Do not be confused by this statement. Your partner must not release manual stabilization of the patient's head until the patient is *fully* immobilized on the spine board.
- To ensure the most appropriately sized cervical collar, measure from the top of the patient's shoulder to just below the earlobe. A collar that is not the correct size will cause either flexion or extension of the patient's neck.

3. Releases or orders the release of manual immobilization before it was maintained mechanically.

- To best avoid making this mistake, tell your partner to maintain manual stabilization of the patient's head and do not allow him or her to release it until after you have completed the application of the cervical immobilization device (CID), which also is referred to as a "head chock."
- Remember, the patient is not considered fully immobilized until he or she is completely secured to the spine board with all straps placed and the CID in place.

4. Manipulates or moves the patient excessively, causing potential spinal compromise.

- Make sure that you inform your partner that no patient moves will take place without his or her command.
- All patient moves, regardless of how slight, must be uniform, and the patient must be moved as a unit at the command of the person maintaining stabilization of the patient's head.
- Should you have to move the spine board to place the straps, make sure that you do this very carefully, without causing the patient to move on the board.

5. Immobilizes the head to the device *before* the device is sufficiently secured to the torso.

- Securing the patient's head to the device prior to securing the torso may cause unnecessary movement of the neck when the straps are applied and secured to the torso and legs.
- Do not mechanically immobilize the head until you have *completely* immobilized the torso. Candidates commonly will position the device in its entirety and then go back and tighten the straps. This is a bad practice that should be avoided.
- It makes no difference whether you immobilize the legs before or after you immobilize the torso; however, *it is critical that the torso is fully immobilized before the head is immobilized.*

6. Device moves excessively up, down, left, or right on the patient's torso.

- To ensure the most effective immobilization of the torso, when placing the patient on the spine board, make sure that he or she is completely centered on the board. Remember, any patient moves must be uniform and at the command of the EMT assistant controlling the head.
- After you have positioned but not secured the torso, step back and look at the patient to make sure that the device is centered, then secure the straps.

7. Head immobilization allows for excessive movement.

- Be sure to use the most appropriately sized cervical collar.
- Make sure that the CID is positioned properly and secured appropriately with one strap placed under the chin of the cervical collar and the other strap over the patient's forehead.

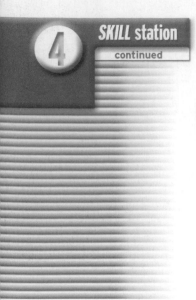

SKILL station
continued

8. **Upon completion of immobilization, head is not in a neutral, in-line position.**
   - Be sure to use the appropriately sized cervical collar, as explained earlier.
   - Make sure that when you are positioning the patient on the spine board, the patient is completely straight prior to immobilizing the head. Unnecessary moves to accomplish this only increase your chance of manipulating the spine.

9. **Failure to reassess motor, sensory, and circulatory functions in *each* extremity after immobilization is complete.**
   - Although you are only required to assess motor, sensory, and circulatory function after you have completed immobilization, you should get into the habit of checking these functions two times. You should check them before you place the cervical collar and then after the patient is fully immobilized to the long spine board.

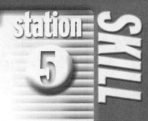
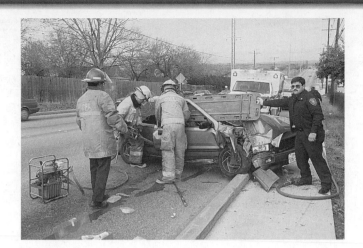

Random Skills

In addition to the five mandatory skills discussed previously, you will be required to perform one skill at random. Prior to successfully completing your initial EMT-Basic training, you had to demonstrate competency in all 13 skills; however, for the Practical Examination, you are only required to perform one of the following skills, which you will not learn of until the day of the exam:

1. Oxygen administration

2. Airway adjuncts and suctioning

3. Mouth-to-mask ventilation with supplemental oxygen

4. Traction splint

5. Immobilization of a joint injury

6. Immobilization of a long bone fracture

7. Bleeding control and shock management

Skill 6A: Oxygen Administration

Station Time Limit: 5 minutes.

Skill Station Objective: This station is designed to test your ability to correctly assemble the equipment needed to administer supplemental oxygen in the prehospital setting. This is an isolated skills test. You will be required to assemble an oxygen tank and regulator and administer oxygen to a patient using a nonrebreathing mask. You will then be instructed to discontinue oxygen therapy with the nonrebreathing mask because the patient cannot tolerate the mask and start oxygen administration using a nasal cannula. Once you have begun oxygen administration using a nasal cannula, you will be instructed to discontinue oxygen administration completely.

Your Partner(s): No EMT assistants are required for this station.

Skill Examiner Function(s): The skill station examiner will track your time during this station, provide you with instructions, and observe your actions.

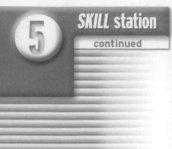

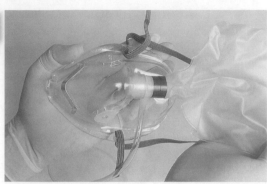

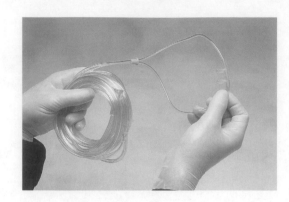

Table 3-7

Oxygen Administration Performance Checklist

Oxygen Administration		
Takes or verbalizes body substance isolation precautions	1	
Assembles the regulator to the tank	1	
Opens tank	1	
Checks for leaks	1	
Checks tank pressure	1	
Attaches nonrebreathing mask to oxygen	1	
Adjusts liter flow to 12 L/min or greater	1	
Prefills reservoir	1	
Applies and adjusts mask to the patient's face	1	
Note: The examiner must advise the candidate that the patient is not tolerating the nonbreathing mask. Medical control has ordered you to apply a nasal cannula to the patient.		
Attaches nasal cannula to oxygen	1	
Adjusts liter flow to 6 L/min or less	1	
Applies nasal cannula to the patient	1	
Note: The examiner must advise the candidate to discontinue oxygen therapy.		
Removes the nasal cannula from the patient	1	
Shuts of the regulator	1	
Relieves the pressure within the regulator	1	
MODELED FROM THE NREMT PERFORMANCE SKILL SHEET	15	

Critical Criteria: Oxygen Administration

1. **Failure to take or verbalize BSI precautions.**
   - So that you do not forget this critical criterion, you might consider physically entering the station with gloves on. The examiner will see this and note that you have taken the appropriate BSI precautions.
2. **Failure to assemble the tank and regulator without leaks.**
   - Be sure that the pin index safety system on the tank is correctly lined up with the corresponding fittings on the regulator.
   - If you turn the oxygen tank on and hear oxygen leaking, simply turn the oxygen off and recheck your fittings.

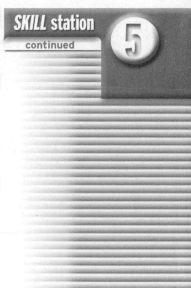
SKILL station
continued
5

3. Failure to adjust the device to the correct liter flow for the nonrebreathing mask (12 L/min or greater).
- You cannot deliver oxygen without making sure the oxygen is flowing. The nonre-breathing mask is capable of delivering up to 90% oxygen. The only way to achieve this is to set the flow rate at 12 L/min or greater.

4. Failure to prefill the reservoir bag.
- The nonrebreathing mask will NOT deliver 100% oxygen if the reservoir is not filled with oxygen. As soon as you set the flowmeter, place your finger over the outlet port within the mask until the reservoir is completely filled.
- *Prior to placing the nonrebreathing mask on the patient,* make sure that the reservoir is completely filled.

5. Failure to adjust the device to the correct liter flow for the nasal cannula (6 L/min or less)
- Prior to placing the nasal cannula on the patient, adjust the liter flow to a range of 1 to 6 L/min.
- The most important aspect to remember is that you must not set the flowmeter to greater than 6 L/min.

Skill 6B: Airway Adjuncts and Suctioning

Station Time Limit: 5 minutes

Skill Station Objective: This station is designed to test your ability to properly measure, insert, and remove an oropharyngeal airway and a nasopharyngeal airway as well as suction the patient's upper airway. This is an isolated skills test composed of three separate skills.

Your Partner(s): No EMT assistants are required for this station.

Skill Examiner Function(s): The skill station examiner will track your time during this station, provide you with instructions, and observe your actions.

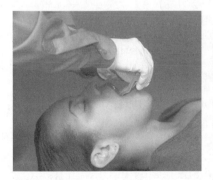
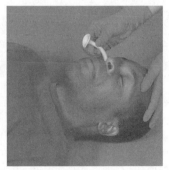
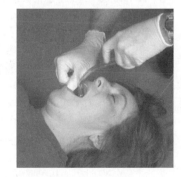

Table 3-8

Airway Adjuncts and Suctioning Performance Checklist

Oropharyngeal Airway		
Takes or verbalizes body substance isolation precautions	1	
Selects appropriately sized airway	1	
Measures airway	1	
Inserts airway without pushing the tongue posteriorly	1	
Note: The examiner must advise the candidate that the patient is gagging and becoming conscious		
Removes oropharyngeal airway	1	
Suction		
Note: The examiner must advise the candidate to suction the patient's oropharynx and nasopharynx		
Turns on and prepares suction device	1	
Ensures presence of mechanical suction	1	
Inserts suction tip without suction	1	
Applies suction to the oropharynx and nasopharynx	1	
Nasopharyngeal Airway		
Note: The examiner must advise the candidate to insert a nasopharyngeal airway.		
Selects appropriately sized airway	1	
Measures airway	1	
Verbalizes lubrication of the nasal airway	1	
Fully inserts the airway with the bevel facing toward the septum	1	
MODELED FROM THE NREMT PERFORMANCE SKILL SHEET	13	

Critical Criteria: Airway Adjuncts and Suctioning

1. Failure to take or verbalize BSI precautions.

- So that you do not forget this critical criterion, you might consider physically entering the station with gloves on. The examiner will see this and note that you have taken the appropriate BSI precautions.

2. Failure to obtain a patent airway with the oropharyngeal airway.

- It is absolutely critical that you select and properly measure for the correctly sized oropharyngeal airway. One that is too small or too large will further occlude the airway.
- The recommended method of measuring for the correctly sized oropharyngeal airway is from the corner of the mouth to the angle of the jaw (or earlobe).
- When the airway is placed properly, the flange should be resting flush with the patient's lips.

3. Failure to obtain a patent airway with the nasopharyngeal airway.

- Again, measuring for the most appropriately sized nasopharyngeal airway is critical.
- The recommended method of measuring for the correctly sized nasopharyngeal airway is from the corner of the nose to the angle of the jaw (or earlobe).
- Do not rotate the airway into place. Simply insert it, with the bevel facing the nasal septum or base of the nostril.
- If you meet resistance, do not force the airway into place. Attempt insertion in the other nostril.

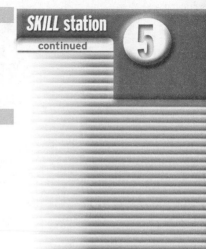

SKILL station
continued
5

4. Failure to demonstrate an acceptable suction technique.
- Measure the suction catheter in the same manner in which you measure the oropharyngeal airway.
- DO NOT suction while inserting the catheter. Suction in a circular motion only while *removing* the catheter from the mouth.
- Suction for no longer than 15 seconds.

5. Inserts any adjunct in a manner dangerous to the patient.
- Examples of a dangerously inserted adjunct include:
  - Forcing an oropharyngeal or nasopharyngeal airway into place.
    - Be sure to lubricate the nasopharyngeal airway.
  - Suctioning while inserting the catheter.
  - Suctioning for longer than 15 seconds.

Skill 6C: Mouth-to-Mask Ventilation with Supplemental Oxygen

Station Time Limit: 5 minutes

Skill Station Objective: This station is designed to test your ability to ventilate a patient with supplemental oxygen using the mouth-to-mask technique. This is an isolated skills test. You may assume that mouth-to-barrier ventilation is in progress and that the patient has a central pulse. The only management required is ventilatory support using the mouth-to-mask technique with supplemental oxygen. You must ventilate the patient for at least 30 seconds. You will be evaluated on the appropriateness of ventilatory volumes.

Your Partner(s): No EMT assistants are required for this station.

Skill Examiner Function(s): The skill station examiner will track your time during this station and observe you for at least 30 seconds, during which time he or she will evaluate the effectiveness of your ventilations.

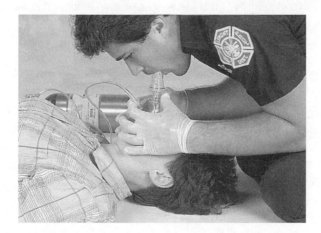

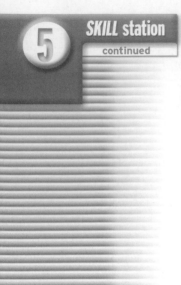

Table 3-9

Mouth-to-Mask Ventilation with Supplemental Oxygen Performance Checklist

Mouth-to-Mask Ventilation with Supplemental Oxygen		
Takes or verbalizes body substance isolation precautions	1	
Connects the one-way valve to the mask	1	
Opens the airway (manually or with an adjunct)	1	
Establishes and maintains a proper mask-to-face seal	1	
Ventilates the patient at the proper volume and rate	1	
Connects the mask to high-concentration oxygen	1	
Adjusts the flow rate to at least 15 L/min	1	
Continues ventilation at proper volume and rate	1	
Note: The examiner must witness ventilations for at least 30 seconds.		
MODELED FROM THE NREMT PERFORMANCE SKILL SHEET	8	

Critical Criteria: Mouth-to-Mask Ventilation with Supplemental Oxygen

1. Failure to take or verbalize BSI precautions.

- So that you do not forget this critical criterion, you might consider physically entering the station with gloves on. The examiner will see this and note that you have taken the appropriate BSI precautions.

2. Failure to adjust liter flow to at least 15 L/min.

- Remember, the objective is to provide ventilations with supplemental oxygen. You can elect to attach the oxygen and set the flowmeter accordingly as soon as you initiate ventilations or you can ventilate with room air and then attach the supplemental oxygen.
- Although a pocket mask without supplemental oxygen will deliver good tidal volume to the patient, it will only deliver 16% oxygen to the patient. With the flowmeter set at 15 L/min, up to 55% oxygen AND good tidal volume can be delivered.

3. Failure to provide proper volume per breath (more than 2 ventilation errors per minute).

- Technique, technique, technique!
- Deliver each breath over 1 second, ensuring that the chest *visibly* rises.
- Use a method of securing the mask to the face that works best for you. Either of the following methods are acceptable, provided that you are able to make the chest *visibly* rise:
  - Kneel at the patient's head, place the mask to the face, grasp the angles of the jaw, and tilt the patient's head back.
  - Kneel astride the patient, perform a head tilt-chin lift maneuver, and place the mask to the patient's face.

4. **Failure to ventilate the patient at a rate of 10 to 12 breaths/min.**
   - This problem is easily avoidable. To achieve a ventilation rate of 10 to 12 breaths/min, ventilate the patient once every 5 to 6 seconds.
   - Count to yourself (or aloud) if you need to in order to ensure the appropriate rate of ventilation.

5. **Failure to allow for complete exhalation.**
   - This happens when you ventilate too fast. **Do not hyperventilate the patient!**
   - Make sure that the chest falls completely prior to initiating another breath.
   - Remember, keep the rate at 10 to 12 breaths/min, and you will be safe.

Skill 6D: Traction Splint

Station Time Limit: 10 minutes

Skill Station Objective: This station is designed to test your ability to properly immobilize a midshaft femoral fracture with a traction splint. You will have an EMT assistant to help you in the application of the device by applying manual traction when directed to do so. You are required to treat only the specific, isolated injury to the femur. Both the scene size-up and initial assessment have been performed, and during the focused assessment, a midshaft femoral deformity was detected. Ongoing assessment of the patient's airway, breathing, and central circulation is not necessary.

Your Partner(s): You will have an EMT assistant who will provide manual traction as you apply the traction device. The EMT assistant will do only what you instruct him or her to do.

Skill Examiner Function(s): The skill station examiner will track your time during this station and observe your actions as well as those of your EMT assistant.

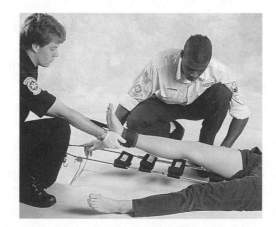

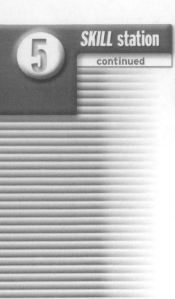

Table 3-10

Traction Splint Performance Checklist

Traction Splint		
Takes or verbalizes body substance isolation precautions	1	
Directs application of manual stabilization of the injured leg	1	
Directs the application of manual traction	1	
Assesses motor, sensory, and distal circulatory function in the injured extremity	1	
Note: The examiner acknowledges that all functions are present and normal.		
Prepares and adjusts splint to the proper length	1	
Positions the splint at the injured leg	1	
Applies the proximal securing device (eg, an ischial strap)	1	
Applies the distal securing device (eg, an ankle hitch)	1	
Applies mechanical traction	1	
Positions and secures the support straps	1	
Reevaluates the proximal and distal securing devices	1	
Reassesses motor, sensory, and distal circulatory function in the injured extremity	1	
Note: The examiner acknowledges that all functions are present and normal.		
Note: The examiner must ask candidate how he or she would prepare the patient for transport.		
Verbalizes securing the torso to the long board to immobilize the hip	1	
Verbalizes securing the splint to the long board to prevent movement of the splint	1	
MODELED AFTER THE NREMT PERFORMANCE SKILL SHEET	14	

Critical Criteria: Traction Splint

1. Loss of traction occurs at any point after it was applied.

- There are two key points that must be addressed so that loss of traction does not occur:
  - Constantly talk with your partner so that there are no "surprise" moves.
  - Make sure that the locking mechanism on the traction splint is truly "locked" after mechanical traction is applied.
- Before your partner assumes manual traction, instruct your partner to place his or her foot against the foot of the patient's uninjured leg. This will prevent the patient from sliding as manual traction is pulled and will allow your partner to maintain his or her balance.

2. Failure to assess motor, sensory, and circulatory function in the injured extremity before and after splinting.

- As soon as you apply manual stabilization to the injured leg, you should immediately assess motor, sensory, and circulatory function. You can also direct your partner to do this.
- Motor, sensory, and circulatory function are then checked after the entire splint has been applied, including mechanical traction.
- Consider checking motor, sensory, and circulatory function three times: after manual stabilization of the leg, after mechanical traction is applied, and after the splint has been completely secured to the patient.

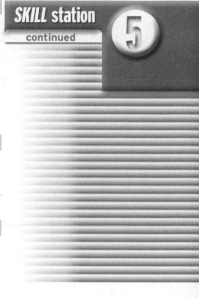

3. The foot was excessively rotated or extended after the splint was applied.
- When preparing the splint for application, compare the splint to the uninjured leg to make sure that the end of the splint extends no more than 12″ beyond the injured leg. This will prevent overextension of the leg once mechanical traction is applied.
- When manually stabilizing the injured leg, make sure that it is as straight as possible and that the foot is pointing straight upward. Maintain this position until application of the splint is completed. This will prevent excessive rotation of the leg.

4. Failure to secure the ischial strap before traction is applied.
- As soon as the traction splint has been placed under the injured leg and you have instructed your partner to lower the leg into the splint, immediately apply the ischial strap. This will secure the traction splint and prevent slipping when mechanical traction is applied.

5. Final immobilization fails to support the femur or prevent rotation of the injured leg.
- Refer to Critical Criteria step 3 regarding prevention of leg rotation.
- Instruct your partner that when you are pulling mechanical traction, he or she must stop you when the amount of mechanical traction meets or slightly exceeds the manual traction he or she is applying. Anything less will cause the leg to "drop" after mechanical traction is applied.
- Make sure that you securely fasten all straps carefully to prevent movement of the leg.

6. Secures the leg to the splint before applying mechanical traction.
- Adequate mechanical traction cannot be applied if the entire splint is secured to the patient's leg first. Remember this general sequence of traction splint application:
  - Apply manual stabilization and check motor, sensory, and circulatory function in the injured leg.
  - Apply the ankle hitch and manual traction.
  - Place the prepared splint under the patient's leg and lower the leg into the splint.
  - Fasten the ischial strap and then apply mechanical traction.
  - Fasten the velcro straps to secure the patient's leg to the splint.
  - Reassess motor, sensory, and circulatory function after complete splint application.
  - Verbalize moving and securing the patient to a long spine board

Note: If the Sager or Kendrick's traction device is used without elevating the patient's leg, application of manual traction is not necessary. The candidate should be awarded 1 point as if manual traction had been applied.

Note: If the leg is to be elevated at all, manual traction must be applied before elevating the leg. The ankle hitch may be applied before elevating the leg and used to provide manual traction.

Skill 6E: Immobilization of a Joint Injury

Station Time Limit: 5 minutes

Skill Station Objective: This station is designed to test your ability to properly immobilize an uncomplicated shoulder injury. You are required to treat only the specific, isolated injury to the shoulder. Both the scene size-up and initial assessment have been performed, and during the focused assessment, a shoulder injury was detected. Ongoing assessment of the patient's airway, breathing, and central circulation is not necessary.

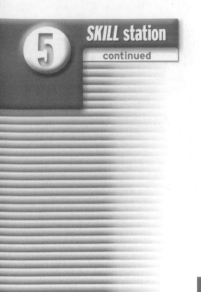

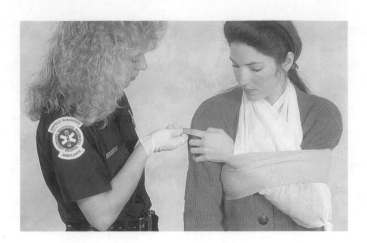

Table 3-11

Joint Immobilization Performance Checklist

Joint Immobilization		
Takes or verbalizes body substance isolation precautions	1	
Directs application of manual stabilization of the shoulder injury	1	
Assesses motor, sensory and distal circulatory function in the injured extremity	1	
Note: The examiner acknowledges that all functions are present and normal.		
Selects proper splinting material	1	
Immobilizes site of the injury	1	
Immobilizes bone above the injured joint	1	
Immobilizes bone below the injured joint	1	
Reassesses motor, sensory, and distal circulatory function in the injured extremity	1	
Note: The examiner acknowledges that all functions are present and normal.		
MODELED FROM THE NREMT PERFORMANCE SKILL SHEET	8	

Your Partner(s): No EMT assistants are required for this skill.

Skill Examiner Function(s): The skill station examiner will track your time during this station and observe your actions. He or she will also check the appropriateness of the immobilization upon completion.

Critical Criteria: Joint Immobilization

1.   Failure to support the joint so that the joint does not bear distal weight.

- When you apply the sling, make sure that the elbow is flexed and the hand is pointing toward the uninjured shoulder. This will allow the elbow of the injured extremity to rest in the sling and provide ample support.
- Use extreme care when applying the sling. You do not want any downward pressure on the injured extremity, which would ultimately cause it to bear distal weight.

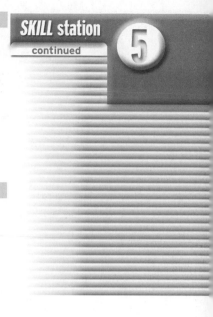

2. Failure to immobilize the bone above and below the injured joint.

- It sometimes can be difficult to determine what bone is proximal to the injured shoulder. Remember that the glenohumeral joint is the most common site for a shoulder dislocation. The glenohumeral joint is where the head of the humerus joins with the glenoid fossa of the scapula. Therefore, the scapula would be the proximal bone that must be immobilized. The sling, when applied and secured properly, will serve this purpose.

- The humerus itself is the distal bone that must be immobilized. The swathe, when applied and secured properly, will serve this purpose. If you feel that another swathe is needed, apply it carefully.

3. Failure to assess motor, sensory, and circulatory functions before and after splinting.

- The first check of motor, sensory, and circulatory function should occur immediately after the injured extremity is manually stabilized. After the sling and swathe are applied, you must again check distal motor, sensory, and circulatory function. Capillary refill will suffice in assessing circulatory function.

Note: In addition to effectively splinting the injured extremity, you must do so without causing further injury. Do not handle the extremity too roughly.

Note: Neatness looks good, but does not count. What counts is effectiveness.

Skill 6F: Immobilization of a Long Bone Fracture

Station Time Limit: 5 minutes

Skill Station Objective: This station is designed to test your ability to properly immobilize a closed, nonangulated long bone injury. Both the scene size-up and initial assessment have been performed, and during the focused assessment, a closed, nonangulated injury of the _____ (radius, ulna, tibia, or fibula) was detected. Ongoing assessment of the patient's airway, breathing, and central circulation is not necessary.

Your Partner(s): No EMT assistants are required for this skill.

Skill Examiner Function(s): The skill station examiner will track your time during this station and observe your actions. He or she will also check the appropriateness of the immobilization upon completion.

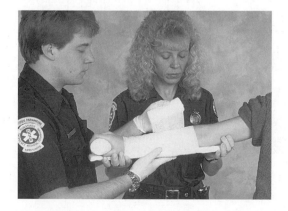

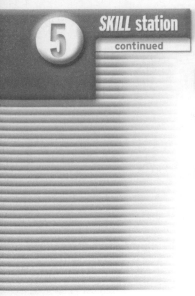

SKILL station
continued

Table 3-12

Immobilization of a Long Bone Fracture Performance Checklist

Long Bone Immobilization		
Takes or verbalizes body substance isolation precautions	1	
Directs application of manual stabilization of the injured extremity	1	
Assesses motor, sensory and distal circulation function in the injured extremity	1	
Note: The examiner acknowledges that all functions are present and normal.		
Measures splint	1	
Applies splint	1	
Immobilizes the joint above the injury site	1	
Immobilizes the joint below the injury site	1	
Secures the entire injured extremity	1	
Immobilizes the hand or foot in the position of function	1	
Reassesses motor, sensory and distal circulation function in the injured extremity	1	
Note: The examiner acknowledges that all functions are present and normal.		
MODELED FROM THE NREMT PERFORMANCE SKILL SHEET	**10**	

Critical Criteria: Immobilization of a Long Bone Fracture

1. Grossly moves the injured extremity.
- First, do no harm. Manually stabilize the injured extremity and do not let go until the entire extremity has been immobilized.
- When applying the splint, allow no sudden movements of the injured extremity. Tell the patient not to move the injured extremity.
- Always use caution.

2. Failure to immobilize the adjacent joints.
- Use this guide to determine what joints must be immobilized, based on the long bone that is injured:
  - Radius or ulna: Immobilize the elbow proximally and the wrist distally.
  - Tibia or fibula: Immobilize the knee proximally and the ankle distally.
- Padded board splints and cravats are most commonly used to immobilize long bone fractures.

3. Failure to assess motor, sensory, and circulatory function before and after splinting.
- The first check of motor, sensory, and circulatory function should occur immediately after the injured extremity is manually stabilized. After the padded board splints or other materials are applied and the injury is completely immobilized, you must again check distal motor, sensory, and circulatory function. Capillary refill will suffice in assessing circulatory function.

Note: In addition to effectively splinting the injured extremity, you must do so without causing further injury. Do not handle the extremity too roughly.

Note: Neatness looks good, but does not count. What counts is effectiveness.

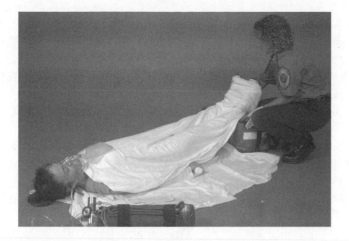

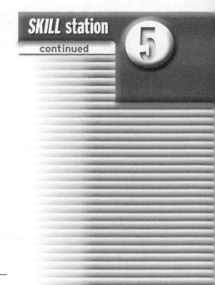

SKILL station
continued
5

Skill 6G: Bleeding Control and Shock Management

Station Time Limit: 10 minutes

Skill Station Objective: This station is designed to test your ability to control hemorrhage. This is a scenario-based testing station. As you progress through the scenario, you will be given various signs and symptoms. A scenario will be read aloud to you and you will be given the opportunity to ask clarifying questions about the scenario; however, you will not receive answers about the actual steps of the procedures to be performed.

Your Partner(s): No EMT assistants are required for this skill.

Skill Examiner Function(s): The skill station examiner will track your time during this station and observe your actions. He or she will provide you with the necessary information so that you may determine the most effective and appropriate treatment.

Table 3-13

Bleeding Control and Shock Management Performance Checklist

Bleeding Control/Shock Management		
Takes or verbalizes body substance isolation precautions	1	
Applies direct pressure to the wound	1	
Elevates the extremity	1	
Applies a dressing to the wound	1	
Bandages the wound	1	
Note: The examiner must now inform the candidate that the wound is still continuing to bleed.		
Applies an additional dressing to the wound	1	
Note: The examiner must now inform the candidate that the wound is still continuing to bleed. The second dressing does not control the bleeding.		
Locates and applies pressure to appropriate arterial pressure point	1	
Note: The examiner must now inform the candidate that the bleeding is controlled and the patient is in compensatory shock.		
Applies a high concentration of oxygen	1	
Properly positions the patient	1	
Initiates steps to prevent heat loss from the patient	1	
Indicates need for immediate transport	1	
MODELED AFTER THE NREMT PERFORMANCE SKILL SHEET	**11**	

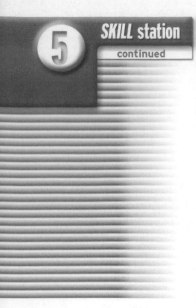

5 *SKILL* station
continued

Critical Criteria: Bleeding Control and Shock Management

1. Failure to take or verbalize body substance isolation precautions.

- So that you do not forget this critical criterion, you might consider physically entering the station with gloves on. The examiner will see this and note that you have taken the appropriate BSI precautions.

2. Failure to apply a high concentration of oxygen.

- Key in on the word "shock." All patients in shock receive 100% oxygen; however, do not set aside prompt bleeding control for this.
- The scenario will start with the assumption that the airway is patent and the patient is breathing adequately.

3. Applies a tourniquet before attempting other methods of bleeding control.

- At this point in your training, it should almost be second nature to slap your gloved hand and dressing on a profound arterial hemorrhage and elevate the extremity at the same time.
- Think about it, how many people have *you* put a tourniquet on because you couldn't stop the bleeding by simpler means?

4. Failure to control hemorrhage in a timely manner.

- Timely means immediately!

5. Failure to indicate a need for immediate transport.

- This will be the last thing that you verbalize.
- Make sure that you do not forget to say "transport."

Summary

Use the information presented in this section to your advantage. Focus on the steps and the critical criteria for each of the covered skills. Frequent practice of not only **what** you are doing, but **why** you are doing it, will greatly enhance your overall performance. Remember that you must be able to be versatile, especially during the patient assessment stations, because the patient's condition frequently changes, requiring you to adjust your thought processes and management accordingly.

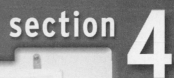

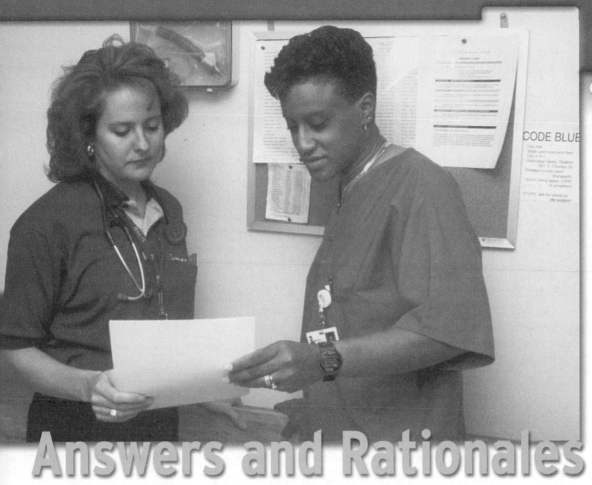

Answers and Rationales

Subtest 1 Practice Exam: Airway and Breathing (25 items)

1. B. In the patient with no trauma, the head tilt-chin lift maneuver is a temporizing measure until an oral or nasal airway adjunct can be inserted to keep the tongue off of the posterior pharynx. You must remember that even once an airway adjunct has been placed, proper positioning of the head must be maintained until the airway is secured more definitively (ie, endotracheal intubation).

2. D. The jaw-thrust maneuver must be used to open the airway any time the mechanism of injury suggests trauma or when the mechanism of injury is unclear (ie, in a patient who became unconscious without witnesses). When performed correctly, the jaw-thrust maneuver maintains a patent airway without manipulating the spine.

3. D. Because this patient was found unconscious next to the bed and his wife did not see what happened, you must assume that the patient fell from the bed and potentially sustained a spinal injury. Because of the potential trauma, the jaw-thrust maneuver must be used, which involves grasping the angles of the lower jaw and lifting forward without manipulating the head. Performing a head tilt-chin lift maneuver could potentially worsen a spinal injury if one exists. After the airway has been opened and cleared if needed, the patient's respirations should be assessed and managed accordingly. This may include applying supplemental oxygen with a nonrebreathing mask or initiating positive pressure ventilations.

4. A. Both inadequate breathing and secretions from the mouth (ie, blood, vomitus, etc) must be addressed simultaneously. This is best accomplished by suctioning in 15-second increments, then providing assisted ventilations for 2 minutes. This pattern must be continued until the airway is clear of secretions. Oral suctioning should not exceed 15 seconds in length. The insertion of an airway adjunct should not occur until the airway is clear of secretions or potential obstructions.

5. A. When ventilating an apneic patient with a bag-valve-mask device, you must ensure that an oral or nasal airway adjunct is inserted, which will keep the tongue off of the posterior pharynx. When ventilating a patient with a BVM device, it is best for you to be positioned at the patient's head to allow for better control of the head. Ventilations in the apneic adult with a pulse (ie, not in cardiac arrest) should be provided at a rate of 10 to 12 breaths/min. Generally, only pediatric sized BVM devices have pop-off relief valves.

6. A. During the active process of inhalation, the muscles of the diaphragm contract, causing the diaphragm to descend. This increases the vertical dimensions of the chest. At the same time, the intercostal muscles (muscles between the ribs) contract, increasing the horizontal dimensions of the chest. These two processes cause intrathoracic pressure to fall, and air rushes in to fill the lungs.

7. C. At the cellular level, oxygen passes across the capillary bed from the arterioles and into the cell, which is facilitated by a process called diffusion, in which oxygen (as any gas) moves from an area of lower concentration to an area of higher concentration. At the same time, carbon dioxide crosses the capillary bed and enters the venule, where it is transported back to the lungs for reoxygenation.

8. B. The preferred method for initially providing artificial ventilations is with the use of a pocket mask attached to supplemental oxygen. Rescuers who ventilate patients infrequently have difficulty maintaining an adequate seal with a BVM device. Because both of the rescuer's hands are freed up when using a pocket mask, it is easier to maintain an adequate seal, thus providing more effective ventilations. The flow-restricted, oxygen-powered ventilatory device requires an oxygen source to function and would thus not be practical as an initial device for providing positive pressure ventilations.

9. C. Unequal or minimal expansion of the chest results in a decrease in the amount of air inhaled per breath (tidal volume). Accessory muscle use and nasal flaring are signs of increased work of breathing. Increases in minute volume result from an increase in tidal volume and/or respiratory rate.

10. A. Signs of inadequate breathing include shallow breathing (reduced tidal volume), a respiratory rate that is too slow (<12 breaths/min) or too fast (>20 breaths/min), an irregular pattern of inhalation and exhalation, and abnormal respiratory sounds (ie, stridor, snoring, wheezing, etc). Even though the patient has a respiratory rate that is within normal limits for an adult, her respirations are shallow (reduced tidal volume). You must evaluate all components of breathing: rate, regularity, depth, and quality.

11. B. In an unresponsive patient, the muscles of the tongue, which attach to the mandible, relax and fall back over the posterior pharynx. This makes obstruction by the tongue the most common cause of airway obstruction in semi- and unconscious patients.

12. C. The airway in unresponsive patients must be protected with an oral or nasal airway adjunct to prevent the tongue from occluding the posterior pharynx. Unresponsive patients who are breathing adequately (good rate, depth, and quality) need 100% supplemental oxygen. The patient must be monitored closely for signs of inadequate breathing, which would require assisted ventilations. Suctioning would be required if the patient had secretions or blood in the airway.

13. A. This patient fell from a significant height and is unresponsive; therefore, initial management consists of opening the patient's airway with the jaw-thrust maneuver. The head tilt-chin lift maneuver would aggravate any possible injuries to the spine that resulted from the fall. After the airway is open, it must be cleared of any secretions. The patient's respirations are then assessed and oxygen is provided via a nonrebreathing mask or assisted ventilations.

14. C. You must assess all parameters of a patient's breathing—rate, regularity, depth, and quality. If a patient's respirations are rapid, you should assess the depth, quality, and regularity of the respirations in order to determine overall breathing adequacy. On the basis of this assessment, the most appropriate management can be delivered—oxygen via a nonrebreathing mask or some form of positive-pressure ventilation (ie, BVM, pocket-mask device). *Adequacy of breathing is not determined by respiratory rate alone.*

15. C. The preferred position of comfort for most patients with respiratory distress is Fowler's position (sitting up). A prone, supine, or lateral recumbent position would make it more difficult for the patient to breathe.

16. B. In order of preference, artificial ventilations should first be attempted with a pocket mask and supplemental oxygen, then the two-person bag-valve-mask technique, a flow-restricted, oxygen-powered ventilation device (FROPVD), and then a one-person bag-valve-mask technique. See rationale #8 for further explanation.

17. A. Tidal volume (V_T) is the amount of air inhaled in a single breath; it is normally 500 mL in the average adult male. Tidal volume is assessed by noting the depth of a patient's respirations. Shallow breathing, for example, would indicate a reduced tidal volume. The volume of air that remains in the upper airway (eg, larger bronchi, trachea) is called dead space volume (V_D); it is approximately 30 percent of the patient's tidal volume and does not participate in pulmonary gas exchange. Therefore, if a patient has a tidal volume of 500 mL, the *actual* volume of air that enters the lungs and participates in gas exchange is 350 mL:

$$500 \text{ mL } (V_T) - 150 \text{ mL } (30\% \text{ of } V_T \text{ } [V_D]) = 350 \text{ mL}$$

The volume of air moved in and out of the lungs per minute is called alveolar minute volume (V_M) and is a computation of the tidal volume (minus dead space volume) multiplied by the respiratory rate. Therefore, if an adult male has a tidal volume of 500 mL and a respiratory rate of 18 breaths/min, his alveolar minute volume would be 6,300 mL:

$$500 \text{ mL } (VT) - 150 \text{ mL } (30\% \text{ of } V_T \text{ } [V_D] \times 18 \text{ (breaths/min)} = 6,300 \text{ mL}$$

The total volume of air that the lungs are capable of holding is called the total lung capacity (TLC), and is approximately 6 L in the average adult male.

18. C. Agonal respirations are occasional, irregular gasping breaths that are commonly seen just before death in patients who are in the midst of complete respiratory failure. Some patients may experience agonal respirations in the first few minutes after their heart has stopped. During the early phases of hypoxia, when the patient is compensating, respirations become rapid (tachypnea) in an attempt to increase the oxygen content of the blood and eliminate more carbon dioxide. However, as the hypoxic patient begins to decompensate, respirations become shallow (reduced tidal volume) and, in some cases, slow (bradypnea). When the tongue partially occludes the airway of a semi- or unconscious patient, a snoring sound is heard.

19. A. Although unlikely, an unconscious patient may have an active gag reflex. If an unconscious patient begins to gag as you are attempting to insert an oropharyngeal airway, you must remove the airway immediately and be prepared to suction if vomiting should occur. Once the airway has been cleared, a nasopharyngeal airway, which is better tolerated in patients with a gag reflex, should be inserted.

20. D. If the patient's chest rises minimally or not at all when you are using the one-person bag-valve-mask technique, you should first reevaluate the mask-to-face seal and make sure that the patient's head is properly positioned. The most common complication associated with the one-person bag-valve-mask technique is difficulty in maintaining an adequate mask-to-face seal. If repositioning does not remedy the problem, you should ensure that you are squeezing the bag hard enough to produce adequate tidal volume. Caution must be used, however, when ventilating a patient; breaths that are delivered too forcefully may cause an increase in intrathoracic pressure, thus impeding blood return to the heart and decreasing cardiac output. Therefore, you should deliver each breath over a period of one second—just enough to produce visible chest rise. The patient's mouth should be suctioned only if it contains secretions or blood.

21. B. When ventilating an adult cardiac arrest patient with an advanced airway in place (ie, ET tube), you should deliver each breath over a period of 1 second—just enough to produce visible chest rise—at a rate of 8 to 10 breaths/min. Do not attempt to synchronize ventilations with chest compressions once the airway has been secured with an advanced device. Hyperventilation should be avoided as it may result in increased intrathoracic pressure and decreased blood return to the heart.

22. A. When ventilating any apneic patient, each breath should be delivered over a period of 1 second—just enough to produce visible chest rise. Excessive ventilation duration and/or volume increases the likelihood of gastric distention—especially if the patient's airway is not secured with an advanced device (ie, ET tube, LMA)—and may result in increased intrathoracic pressure, decreased venous return to the heart, and decreased cardiac output.

23. A. Although the patient is restless—a sign of hypoxemia—she is conscious and alert and able to maintain her own airway; therefore, an airway adjunct is not needed at this point. Furthermore, her respirations, although increased in rate, are producing adequate tidal volume as evidenced by adequate chest expansion. Therefore, she is not in need of ventilatory assistance at this point. The most appropriate airway management would be to administer 100% oxygen with a nonrebreathing mask and closely monitor her for signs of inadequate breathing (ie, shallow breathing [reduced tidal volume], decreased level of consciousness, cyanosis, etc). A nasal cannula is not an appropriate oxygen delivery device to use in an acutely hypoxemic patient.

24. **A.** Before breathing can be assessed, let alone managed, the airway must be cleared of any and all secretions. When you hear gurgling respirations, you should provide immediate suctioning of the oropharynx for up to 15 seconds and then provide the appropriate oxygenation, which in this patient would be assisted ventilations. Suctioning in 15-second increments should be provided as needed, followed by assisted ventilations for 2 minutes. This pattern should be repeated until the airway is clear of secretions.

25. **D.** Wheezing is a whistling sound that results from narrowing of the bronchioles in the lungs and thus indicates a lower airway disease (ie, asthma, bronchitis, etc). Crowing and stridor are both high-pitched sounds that indicate an upper airway disease or obstruction, and gurgling indicates secretions in the oropharynx.

Subtest 2 Practice Exam: Cardiology (25 items)

1. **C.** An irregular pulse signifies an abnormality within the electrical conduction system of the heart. Tachycardia, sudden fainting (syncope), and tachypnea (rapid breathing) can indicate many things other than cardiac problems, such as shock, heat-related problems, and diabetic complications. You should always consider the potential for cardiac compromise in a patient with an irregular pulse.

2. **B.** Oxygen is the first and most important therapy for any patient with potential cardiac compromise and should be given without delay. After applying oxygen, you should perform a focused history and physical exam and obtain baseline vital signs. You would inquire about any prescription medications the patient is taking (eg, NTG) during the SAMPLE history.

3. **B.** Whether a patient is found unconscious or loses consciousness in your presence, the first step is to open and maintain the airway. Further management is based on your initial assessment findings and may include attaching an AED if the patient is in cardiac arrest.

4. **C.** The pulmonary vein is the only vein that carries oxygen-rich blood. It carries blood from the lungs back to the left atrium. All other veins in the human body, including the vena cava, carry deoxygenated blood back to the heart. The aorta is the largest artery in the body and branches immediately from the left ventricle, carrying freshly oxygenated blood to the rest of the body. The pulmonary artery carries deoxygenated blood from the right ventricle to the lungs for reoxygenation.

5. **D.** According to the 2005 Emergency Cardiac Care (ECC) guidelines, the AED can safely be used in children between 1 and 8 years of age. You should use pediatric pads and a dose-attenuating system (energy reducer); however, if these features are not available, a regular AED should be used. The AED should only be applied to patients in cardiac arrest; if a patient is at risk for cardiac arrest, have the AED ready but not applied. The AED will not analyze the cardiac rhythm if the patient is moving (ie, CPR is in progress). AEDs can be used in patients with implanted pacemakers; ensure that the pads are at least 1" away from the pacemaker.

6. A. Nitroglycerin is a smooth muscle relaxant. Smooth muscle is found within the walls of the blood vessels. Nitroglycerin causes vasodilation, including dilation of the coronary arteries, which in turn allows more blood supply to the heart, increasing the oxygen supply to the heart. However, care must be taken when administering nitroglycerin to a patient. Because of its vasodilatory effects, nitroglycerin can cause the patient's blood pressure to drop. Nitroglycerin should not be administered to patients with a systolic blood pressure of less than 100 mm Hg.

7. C. Once you have determined that a patient is in cardiac arrest, you should immediately begin CPR and prepare the AED for use. Once the AED is ready, you should immediately apply it to the patient and analyze his or her cardiac rhythm. Management of the airway should take place after the AED has been attached, the cardiac rhythm analyzed, and a shock delivered (if indicated). After the AED has delivered a shock, immediately resume CPR, obtain a SAMPLE history from the patient's wife, and notify medical control as needed.

8. C. When performing two-rescuer adult CPR, you should perform "cycles" of CPR, with a compression to ventilation ratio of 30:2. If the airway is not secured with an advanced device (ie, ET tube) ventilations and chest compressions should be coordinated (synchronous). After your partner delivers 30 compressions, ask him or her to pause as you deliver two ventilations. All contact with the patient must cease as the AED is analyzing the cardiac rhythm. When performing chest compressions on an adult, you should "push hard and fast", compressing the chest to a depth of 1 ½" to 2".

9. A. The AED should remain attached to the patient during transport in case he goes back into cardiac arrest while you are en route to the hospital. If this occurs, you should immediately tell your partner to stop the ambulance and assist you in the back as you begin CPR. Remember that the AED will not analyze the cardiac rhythm if the patient is moving. Once your partner is available to assist, you should analyze the cardiac rhythm and defibrillate if indicated. Medical control should be contacted as soon as it is feasible, but not prior to defibrillating the patient.

10. B. You should apply 100% oxygen and provide transport to the hospital without delay to any patients who report chest pain and do not have prescribed nitroglycerin. An EMT-B who knowingly administers someone else's medication to a patient could be held negligent. Medical control should always be contacted when in doubt. However, bear in mind that medical control will not allow you to assist a patient with someone else's medication. The AED is not applied to patients who are breathing and have a pulse.

11. C. The most common cause of cardiac arrest in the adult population is a cardiac arrhythmia—usually ventricular fibrillation—in up to 70% of cases. This fact underscores the importance of early defibrillation to shock the heart back into a perfusing rhythm. According to the American Heart Association, cardiac arrest—again, most often the result of an arrhythmia—occurs in up to 40% of patients experiencing an acute myocardial infarction (AMI). The risk of cardiac arrest is highest within the first 4 hours following the onset of an AMI. Respiratory failure is the most common cause of cardiac arrest in children, not adults. Children generally have healthy hearts and uncommonly experience cardiac arrest due to a primary cardiac event.

12. C. The pain associated with cardiac compromise most commonly is described as pressure, crushing pain, or a sensation of heaviness. However, you should not rule out a cardiac problem just because the patient does not have the "classic" quality of pain.

13. B. If the AED advises you not to shock, you should first check the patient for a pulse because the patient may now have one. If a pulse is absent, immediately resume CPR and reanalyze the cardiac rhythm after 2 minutes of CPR.

14. A. The aorta, which is the largest artery in the human body, originates immediately from the left ventricle where it branches into the coronary arteries. This allows the myocardium to receive blood that has the highest concentration of oxygen. The superior and inferior venae cavae return oxygen-poor blood from the systemic circulation back to the right atrium, where it is pumped into the right ventricle. The left atrium receives freshly oxygenated blood from the lungs.

15. C. According to the American Heart Association, when EMS arrives more than 4 to 5 minutes after being dispatched, a brief period of CPR (1 1/2 to 3 minutes) before defibrillation has been shown to improve return of spontaneous circulation (ROSC) and survival rates in adult patients with unwitnessed cardiac arrest. In cases where the patient's cardiac arrest is witnessed, an AED should be applied without delay. Because cardiac arrest secondary to trauma is usually the result of massive blood loss or other mortal injuries, defibrillation is unlikely to have a positive effect. The patient's past medical history has no effect on whether to perform CPR first or defibrillate first.

16. C. Because nitroglycerin causes vasodilation, including of the vessels within the brain, the cranium is engorged with blood. This causes a pounding headache for the patient. As uncomfortable as it is for the patient, headaches are a normal and expected side effect of the drug. The vasodilatory effects of nitroglycerin could result in hypotension. Therefore, the patient's blood pressure should be carefully monitored. Nausea and anxiety are common symptoms of cardiac compromise, not nitroglycerin.

17. B. Nitroglycerin should be administered to patients who have the prescribed drug with them, a systolic blood pressure of greater than 100 mm Hg, and have not exceeded the maximum recommended dose of three tablets or sprays. An expired medication should never be administered to any patient, even if the drug is indicated.

18. C. The left ventricle is the most powerful chamber of the heart. It does most of the work; therefore, it has the thickest walls. A palpable pulse represents left ventricular contraction. Because the left ventricle does most of the work for the heart, it has an extremely high oxygen demand. This makes it the most common site for a heart attack (myocardial infarction).

19. B. In addition to increasing the body's oxygen supply with 100% supplemental oxygen, it is extremely important to decrease oxygen demand. You can most effectively accomplish this by keeping the patient calm, providing reassurance, and providing safe, prompt transport to the hospital. Traveling at a high rate of speed with lights flashing and siren blasting would clearly increase the patient's anxiety and the heart's demand for oxygen. The decision to request ALS support is based on the patient's condition.

20. A. When questioning any patient about any type of pain, you should avoid asking leading questions that can simply be answered yes or no. To obtain the most reliable assessment, open-ended questions should be asked to allow the patient to describe the quality of the pain in his or her own words.

21. **D.**   When performing CPR on any patient, you should allow the chest to fully recoil after each compression. Incomplete chest recoil causes increased intrathoracic pressure with subsequent decreases in coronary and cerebral perfusion. A pulse should be assessed after 5 cycles (about 2 minutes) of CPR. A compression to ventilation ratio of 30:2 should be performed during one-rescuer CPR (adult, child, and infant), except for newborns. A compression to ventilation ratio of 15:2 is used during two-rescuer infant and child CPR. Ventilations should be delivered over a period of 1 second each; this will minimize the incidence of gastric distention.

22. **C.**   After you have performed the initial assessment of a patient and initiated treatment, your partner should obtain a set of baseline vital signs, which includes measuring the blood pressure. After the vital signs are obtained, the SAMPLE history is obtained, which includes gathering the patient's medications. Once you have completed your assessment, including obtaining the vital signs and SAMPLE history, you should contact medical control if guidance is needed.

23. **B.**   An important aspect of managing a patient with chest pain is to ensure that the patient is in a comfortable position. Most of the time, the patient will already be in this position upon your arrival. A position of comfort will aid in minimizing anxiety, which in turn decreases cardiac oxygen demand. After you make sure that the patient is in a comfortable position, you should administer 100% oxygen. Following assessment, if you feel that ALS support is needed, you should request it. If the patient has prescribed, unexpired nitroglycerin, the systolic blood pressure is greater than 100 mm Hg, and the patient has not taken the maximum of three doses, you should contact medical control to obtain permission to assist the patient in taking the nitroglycerin.

24. **B.**   With tachycardia, as the heart beats faster, it demands more oxygen. Tachycardia can be extremely detrimental to the patient with a compromised heart that is already deprived of oxygen. Keeping the patient calm cannot be overemphasized. The more anxious the patient gets, the faster the heart will beat.

25. **C.**   Information obtained at the scene—whether from first responders or family members—is not always accurate. If the AED advises you to defibrillate, you should do so and then immediately begin or resume CPR. During CPR, ensure adequate oxygenation and ventilation, minimize interruptions in chest compressions, obtain the patient's medical history if possible, and contact medical control as needed. At no time during resuscitative efforts should you detach the AED from the patient. Reanalyze the patient's cardiac rhythm after 2 minutes of CPR and follow the voice prompts.

Subtest 3 Practice Exam: Trauma (25 items)

1. **C.**   The patient's mental status provides you with the most information regarding overall perfusion status, especially when monitoring a patient with a head injury. Frequent neurologic assessments are critical to determine if the patient's condition is improving or getting worse. Vital signs should be monitored according to the patient's condition.

2. **A.**   The radius and ulna are the bones of the forearm. The radial pulse can be palpated on the lateral aspect (thumb side) of the wrist and is the most distal pulse site relative to the injury. The brachial pulse is located on the medial aspect of the upper arm. The popliteal pulse is located behind the knee. The pedal pulse is located on top of the foot.

3. A. It is clear that this patient's airway is patent, as evidenced by his screaming. Blood spurting from the groin area indicates arterial bleeding from the femoral artery. If this bleeding is not controlled immediately, the patient will die. Oxygen and other shock management treatments must be initiated after this life-threatening bleeding is controlled. If you take the time to set up and administer oxygen prior to managing the bleeding, the patient will die. Treatment must be based on what is going to kill the patient *first*.

4. C. Injuries to the shoulder are most effectively immobilized with the use of a sling and swathe. The sling will provide support and relieve pain to the shoulder, and the swathe will secure the arm to the body. The purpose of the swathe is not to facilitate traction. Patients with dislocated or fractured shoulders will not allow you to extend their arm, so any attempt to immobilize the injury in such a fashion will not be possible and could worsen the injury.

5. B. Significant mechanisms of injury include, among others, falls of greater than 15′ (or three times the adult patient's height), penetrating injuries to the trunk and head, high-speed motor vehicle crashes, rollover motor vehicle crashes, ejection from a motor vehicle, and motor vehicle crashes in which another person in the same passenger compartment was killed. In cases such as this, you must assume that the same violent forces that killed the passenger were sustained by the patient, regardless of whether the patient is stable or not.

6. B. Your patient's Glasgow Coma Scale (GCS) score is 7. He gets 2 points for opening his eyes in response to pain, 2 points for speaking with incomprehensible words, and 3 points for withdrawing from pain with flexor (decorticate) posturing. The GCS is a valuable neurologic assessment tool; it should be reassessed frequently in seriously injured patients—especially patients with a head injury.

7. B. After ensuring a patent airway, you must assess the respirations for rate, depth, and quality to determine what airway management is most appropriate for the patient. Remember the mnemonic "OCAM," which stands for open the airway, clear the airway of any secretions, assess the respirations, and manage the airway accordingly. After the airway has been managed, the patient's circulation should be assessed. Assessing the patient's skin condition can be accomplished at the same time you assess the radial and carotid pulses.

8. C. During both the general impression and the initial assessment, you should assess for major bleeding. If there is no obvious bleeding, you would continue your assessment as usual. It is during the rapid trauma assessment, when log rolling the patient to assess the posterior, that you would be most likely to find a small caliber gunshot wound, especially if there is little or no bleeding.

9. A. The goal of managing a sucking chest wound (open pneumothorax) is to prevent air from entering the wound and then reassess the patient's ventilatory status. This is most effectively accomplished by applying an occlusive dressing or similar material to the wound. A porous trauma dressing will not provide the occlusive effect that you need. Three sides of the dressing should be secured and the patient continuously monitored. If the patient begins to exhibit signs of worsened respiratory distress and shock, a tension pneumothorax is most likely developing, and you must release pressure from the thoracic cavity by lifting up the unsecured portion of the occlusive dressing.

10. B. When you apply a vest-style immobilization device such as a KED, you must immobilize the patient's head after the torso is secured. If you immobilize the head first, the cervical spine may be unnecessarily manipulated as you secure the torso. Prior to securing the torso straps, you should ask the patient to inhale as much as possible so that when the straps are secured, enough space is allowed for the patient to breathe adequately. After full immobilization, the patient's spine should be completely in-line, from the head to the pelvis. During the entire immobilization procedure, the patient's head must be maintained in a neutral in-line position.

11. B. During shock, the compensatory mechanisms of the body attempt to maintain the blood pressure. This is accomplished by increases in heart rate, shunting of blood from the skin to more vital organs, and increasing the respiratory rate to increase the oxygen content of the blood. Once these compensatory mechanisms are no longer able to sustain the patient, the blood pressure will fall. This signifies a state of decompensated shock. You must not rely on the patient's blood pressure as an indicator of overall perfusion. Restlessness, anxiety, tachycardia, and cool clammy skin (diaphoresis) are earlier signs of shock and do not necessarily indicate a decompensated state.

12. C. General care for an amputated body part includes wrapping the part in a moist, sterile dressing and keeping it cool. Placing the wrapped part in a plastic bag and putting it on ice can accomplish this. The amputated part must never be placed directly on ice because this will cause cell and tissue damage. Attempting to clean the amputated part or immersing it directly in water can also cause further cell and tissue damage.

13. A. Generally, impaled objects should be stabilized in place and not removed; however, if they interfere with the patient's airway or your ability to perform CPR, they must be carefully removed. The knife in this patient is impaled in the area where chest compressions must be performed (precordium). The AED is not indicated for victims of traumatic cardiac arrest. Blood loss is the most common cause of traumatic cardiac arrest and, therefore, the AED would not be of benefit.

14. B. Unless there is an immediate threat to your or the patient's life, you should apply an extrication collar, slide a long spine board under the patient's buttocks, turn and place the patient on the board, and remove the patient from the car during a rapid extrication. You must be careful to control the cervical spine at all times during extrication. A vest-style extrication device would not be appropriate for a rapid extrication because it takes too long to apply. An emergency move would necessitate removing the patient from the car without any immobilization equipment.

15. A. When assessing the chest during the rapid trauma assessment, you should check for symmetry (equal rise of the chest), assess for pain upon palpation and the presence of equal breath sounds bilaterally. Crepitus also should be noted if present. Rigidity, guarding, and distention should be assessed for when evaluating the abdomen.

16. D. Management of an open abdominal wound with an eviscerated bowel includes controlling any external bleeding, covering the exposed bowel with a moist, sterile dressing, and covering that with a dry, sterile dressing. Applying a dry dressing directly to the exposed bowel will cause the bowel to dry. You must never replace the exposed bowel into the abdominal cavity or apply pressure to the wound. Doing so significantly increases the patient's risk for infection as well as further trauma.

17. C. The goal of the initial assessment is to identify and manage all life-threatening injuries. In the case of this patient, as your partner provides in-line cervical spine control and simultaneously initiates the appropriate airway management, you must take steps to control the bleeding. Typically, your partner will be responsible for managing the airway as you assess and treat other life threats. Most EMS systems work with two-person crews and do not have the luxury of a third EMT. If the police or fire department is on the scene, you can ask them to gather equipment for you. The request for an ALS ambulance is based on factors such as the patient's condition and transport time to the closest appropriate hospital.

18. A. Using the adult Rule of Nines, the anterior trunk (chest and abdomen) accounts for 18% of the body surface area (BSA) and each entire arm accounts for 9%. Therefore, the anterior chest, which is one half of the trunk, would account for 9% BSA, and both anterior arms (4.5% each) would account for 9% BSA, for a total of 18% BSA burned.

19. C. After moving the patient to safety, stopping the burning process, and appropriately supporting the ABCs, full-thickness burns are cared for by applying dry, sterile dressings or burn pads and preventing hypothermia. You should never cool a full-thickness burn in the field because it increases the risk for hypothermia. Rings, necklaces, and other potentially constrictive devices should be removed in the event severe swelling occurs. If portions of clothing are adhered to the skin, they should not be peeled away from the body, but cut around, to prevent further soft-tissue damage.

20. B. Care for any soft-tissue injury begins with controlling any external bleeding. Once bleeding control is accomplished, distal circulation, motor, and sensory functions should be checked, the wound dressed and bandaged, and then distal circulation, motor, and sensory functions rechecked. The injured area can be immobilized as well to prevent further injury. Generally, open wounds are not cleaned in the field.

21. D. Patients with significant head injury must be managed with immobilization of the spine, 100% supplemental oxygen, or assisted ventilations and should be continuously monitored for vomiting. Elevation of the foot of the spine board may cause more blood to engorge the brain, which will increase intracranial pressure (ICP). You should never attempt to control bleeding from the ears of a patient with a head injury because this too will result in increased ICP. If a patient with an isolated head injury begins showing signs of shock (ie, tachycardia, diaphoresis, tachypnea, etc), you should manage the patient as though there is internal bleeding, which would include elevating the lower extremities and preventing the loss of body heat.

22. D. Basic shock management, which should be initiated as soon as possible, includes applying 100% oxygen, elevating the lower extremities 6″ to 12″, and providing warmth. Pneumatic antishock garments are not routinely used for patients in shock unless the shock is associated with an unstable pelvis or multiple lower extremity fractures. Elevation of the upper body in a patient with shock will decrease blood flow to the brain.

23. D. When small blood vessels beneath the skin are damaged, blood seeps into the soft tissues. This manifests as a bruise, also referred to as ecchymosis. A hematoma develops when larger blood vessels are ruptured and the internal bleeding forms a "lump." Cyanosis is a blue-grayish discoloration of the skin and signifies a lack of oxygen in the blood. Mottling occurs when the skin takes on a blotched, purplish appearance and is a sign of shock (hypoperfusion).

24. C. When assessing a patient who has sustained a gunshot wound, you should routinely look for an exit wound, which may be difficult to find. Exit wounds can be a source of continued bleeding, both externally and internally. They may or may not follow the same path as the entrance wound. This is why it is important to conduct a thorough examination of the patient. Ice can be applied to the wound, but only after the wound has been covered by a sterile dressing. Determining why the patient was shot is the responsibility of law enforcement, not the EMT-B. If the wound is close to an extremity, pulse, motor, and sensory function should be assessed distal to the wound.

25. B. In the early stages of shock, hypoxia to the brain causes the patient to become restless and anxious. As shock progresses, the pulse becomes thready (weak), signifying a falling blood pressure, and the patient eventually loses consciousness. It is critical to recognize the early signs of shock and initiate immediate care and rapid transport. You should not rely on the blood pressure as an indicator of perfusion in any patient.

Subtest 4 Practice Exam: Medical (25 items)

1. A. When caring for a patient with an emotional or psychiatric crisis, your primary concern is for your own personal safety as well as your partner's. Your ultimate goal is to get the patient to the hospital safely. Keep in mind that patients with emotional problems may appear calm initially; however, there is always the potential for them to turn violent.

2. C. Diabetic coma (hyperglycemic ketoacidosis) is characterized by a severely high blood glucose level; slow onset; warm, dry skin (from dehydration); and Kussmaul's respirations, which are deep and rapid and have a fruity or acetone odor. Insulin shock results from a low blood glucose level and is characterized by a rapid onset and cool, clammy skin.

3. B. When assessing a patient who has taken an overdose of a medication, you should first ask what was ingested, which will provide you with immediate information about whether or not the substance is toxic. You should then find out when the medication was ingested. This information will provide medical control with the information needed to direct the most appropriate treatment. The patient's weight also should be estimated in kilograms in the event that an antidote is required. Obtaining a history of prior substance abuse can be obtained in the focused physical exam.

4. A. The nature of illness is a category in which you place the patient based on the chief complaint. A chief complaint of confusion and incoherent speech suggests that altered mental status is the nature of illness. An altered mental status can encompass a variety of problems, including diabetic and behavioral problems. This patient's chief complaint is not consistent with cardiac compromise.

5. A. This patient is experiencing a severe allergic reaction (anaphylaxis). Stridor, which is a high-pitched sound heard on inhalation, represents swelling of the structures and tissues of the upper airway and indicates progressive airway closure.

6. B. Assessment of a patient's abdomen includes asking where the pain is located and then palpating that area last. Palpating the painful area first will interfere with the rest of your assessment because of the significant pain the patient will be in. Bowel sounds are of little to no value in the field and generally are not included in the abdominal assessment. Patients with abdominal pain typically prefer to lie on their side with their knees drawn up into their chest. Moving them from this position will aggravate their pain.

7. A. Any type of bright light, especially if shone directly into the eyes, will cause the patient with a headache unnecessary severe pain. Dimming the lights and making the patient as comfortable as possible are the treatments of choice for a patient with a headache. Oxygen also should be administered as needed. Typically, the patient will prefer to lie supine or on the side. Vital signs should be monitored based on the patient's condition.

8. C. Unilateral weakness (weakness on one side of the body) is a significant finding in a patient with a headache because it could indicate a stroke. Abdominal, chest, and leg pain are not common complaints associated with a headache.

9. A. Weight loss, fever, and night sweats indicate both tuberculosis and HIV/AIDS; however, the purplish lesions on the skin, which are called Kaposi's sarcoma, are malignant skin tumors and are a classic finding in patients in the later stages of AIDS.

10. B. Care for a patient with a bite from a pit viper (rattlesnake, copperhead, and water moccasin) includes keeping the patient calm, administering 100% oxygen, keeping the affected part below the level of the heart, and immobilizing it. Never apply ice to a snakebite or the blood vessels will constrict and force the venom deeper into the patient's circulation. If a constricting band is applied, it should be proximal to the bite and should be tight enough to slow venous return only, not cut off arterial supply.

11. B. Seizure deaths are most frequently the result of hypoxia; therefore, your primary focus for a patient who is having a seizure should be on ensuring effective ventilation. Many patients who are having seizures are not breathing adequately and will require assisted ventilation. Secretions from the mouth should be suctioned as needed. Other measures include protecting the patient from injury, avoiding restraining the patient, and not attempting to pry open the patient's mouth.

12. D. Often, an altered mental status can be difficult to assess, especially if you do not know how the patient normally acts. However, there are key findings that should increase your index of suspicion. An abnormal speech pattern, such as slurring or incoherent words, can be the result of a diabetic problem, alcohol intoxication, or drug ingestion. All of these can cause an altered mental status. The presence of medication bottles alone or a patient whose eyes are closed or who appears tired does not indicate an altered mental status.

13. B. Your first action in a heat-related emergency is to move the patient to a cooler environment. Once you have moved the patient to a cooler place, you should begin your assessment and treat the patient accordingly.

14. A. Because the patient has hot, moist skin and an altered mental status, you should suspect the patient is experiencing heatstroke, the most lethal of all heat-related emergencies. Although hot, dry skin is a classic finding in heatstroke, it is not always seen. The fact that the patient is semiconscious and his skin is "hot" is consistent with heatstroke.

15. C. The hypothalamus, which is located within the brain stem, regulates body temperature and acts as the thermostat for the body. In heat-related emergencies, the hypothalamus can "reset" from the normal 98.6°F to a much higher temperature in response to the external environment and the body's inability to release heat.

16. C. Patients with severe hypothermia (body temperature <86°F) who are in cardiac arrest should be managed with basic life support (chest compressions and ventilations), passive external rewarming (ie, removal of wet clothing, applying warm blankets), and rapid transport to the hospital where they can be actively rewarmed. Because cold muscle is a poor conductor of electricity, defibrillation, if indicated, should be limited to 1 attempt until the patient's body temperature has been increased. Cold muscle is a poor conductor of electricity and most likely will not respond to defibrillation.

17. A. When dealing with a psychiatric patient who is silent and unwilling to speak to you, do not fear the silence. The patient simply does not wish to speak. You should not press the issue, for doing so may upset the patient. You should remain calm until the patient speaks to you, and then respond accordingly.

18. A. When a patient falls into the water or becomes panicked when in the water, he or she begins to swallow large amounts of water. Even a small amount of water near the larynx can cause a spasm, which closes off the airway. This results in hypoxia and subsequent loss of consciousness. If the patient is not removed from the water at once, the laryngospasm will relax, and water will fill the lungs.

19. A. Frostbitten extremities should not be rewarmed if there is a chance that they could refreeze after you have rewarmed them. Refreezing of an extremity will cause further or worsened tissue and cellular damage. A delay in getting the patient to the emergency department warrants rewarming. If rewarmed, the extremity should be immersed in water that is 105° to 112°F. Analgesia would certainly be a comfort to the patient, but is not mandatory for the rewarming process.

20. B. Hydrocodone (Vicodin) is a potent narcotic (opiate) drug that suppresses the central nervous system, thus depressing respirations, heart rate, and blood pressure. Initial management of any patient who has taken an overdose of a medication of this type is to support breathing. Because this patient is breathing inadequately, immediate assisted ventilations are needed. You also should consider requesting an ALS ambulance if transport time to the nearest hospital will be lengthy. Paramedics can administer a drug called naloxone (Narcan) to reverse the effects of narcotic drugs.

21. C. Narcotic (opiate) medication overdoses cause the pupils to become constricted (pinpoint). Barbiturates typically cause pupillary dilation. Because narcotics are central nervous system depressants, you can expect to see hypotension and a decreased tidal volume (shallow breathing) secondary to respiratory depression.

22. A. Propoxyphene (Darvon) is in the narcotic (opiate) class of drugs. Other narcotics include heroin, morphine, codeine, and meperidine (Demerol). Phenobarbitol is an example of a barbiturate. Drugs such as Valium and Xanax are benzodiazepines. Amphetamines include drugs such as Ritalin and Adderall.

23. B. Without knowing if and when the patient last took her insulin, it is difficult to determine if she is experiencing diabetic coma or insulin shock. Nonetheless, her rapid, shallow respirations—which are likely not producing adequate tidal volume—must be treated with ventilation assistance. Because she is unconscious and obviously unable to swallow, oral glucose is contraindicated. If the patient is experiencing diabetic coma, insulin is what she truly needs; however, insulin is typically not administered in the prehospital setting—even by paramedics. After ensuring adequate oxygenation and ventilation, you must transport this patient rapidly to the hospital for definitive treatment.

24. C. If a violent patient needs to be restrained, you must ensure the presence of at least four people (one per extremity). One of the EMTs must continuously talk to the patient to explain what is happening. Restraint is a last resort used to protect the EMT as well as the patient. Consent is not needed from a family member prior to restraining the patient. Just enough force to effectively restrain the patient is all that is required to prevent causing unnecessary injury.

25. C. The liver and gallbladder lie within the right upper quadrant of the abdomen. Most of the stomach is within the left upper quadrant, as is the entire spleen.

Subtest 5 Practice Exam: Obstetrics and Pediatrics (25 items)

1. C. Seizures in children most often are the result of fever (febrile seizures). The occurrence of seizures is not necessarily affected by how high the child's fever gets, but how quickly it rises. The hypothalamus in the brain may not be able to accommodate such abrupt increases in body temperature. High fevers in children can be the result of massive infections, such as meningitis or encephalitis.

2. C. After ensuring an open and clear airway, it is extremely important to keep the newborn warm. Newborns cannot maintain body temperature very well and hypothermia can develop very quickly. Free-flow (blow-by) oxygen should be initiated if the newborn is breathing adequately but has cyanosis to the face, neck, or trunk (central cyanosis). The umbilical cord should not be clamped and cut until the cord has stopped pulsating and the baby is breathing adequately.

3. C. The responding EMT must handle cases of suspected child abuse delicately. You must never accuse the parents or caregiver of abuse. If you are wrong, you could be held liable for slander. Actions that would suggest such accusation includes summoning the police to have the parents arrested. Instead, you must advise the parents or caregiver that the child needs to be transported by ambulance, even if the injury is not life threatening. The goal is to get the child to safety; however, this must be done legally (with parental consent). Once at the hospital, you must apprise the physician of your suspicions.

4. C. When assessing a patient in labor, the first question you should ask is how far along in the pregnancy she is. If she is at less than 37 weeks' gestation, you should prepare for possible resuscitation of the newborn if delivery occurs in the field. Other questions, such as asking if her amniotic sac (bag of waters) has ruptured and whether or not she has received prenatal care also can help you anticipate and prepare for potential complications. You should also inquire as to how many times the patient has been pregnant (gravida) and the number of times she has delivered a viable newborn (para).

5. D. When crowning occurs, which clearly is a delivery in progress, you should apply gentle pressure to the infant's head to prevent an explosive delivery. Care must be taken to avoid putting pressure on the fontanels (the soft spots on the infant's head). Crowning represents the end of the first stage of labor and the beginning of the second stage and does not always occur immediately after the amniotic sac has ruptured. If the infant's head is born and the amniotic sac is still intact, you need to pinch the thin membrane with your fingers, which will usually cause the sac to easily rupture.

6. B. If, during transport, the mother begins to deliver the infant, your first action should be to advise your partner to stop the ambulance and assist you with the delivery. Delivery of a baby should never be attempted in the back of a moving ambulance.

7. A. Positive pressure ventilations are indicated in the newborn if the heart rate falls to less than 100 beats/min or if central cyanosis persists despite the delivery of blow-by (free-flow) oxygen. Chest compressions are indicated if the heart rate is less than 60 beats/min.

8. B. Limb presentations represent a dire emergency for the newborn and do not spontaneously deliver in the field. You must place the mother in a head-down position with her hips elevated in an attempt to slide the infant slightly back into the birth canal and remove pressure from the umbilical cord. Both 100% oxygen for the mother and immediate transport are indicated.

9. B. Following a sexual assault of a woman, it is not at all uncommon for the patient to not want a member of the opposite sex to touch her. The EMT-B must be very sensitive to this. If a female EMT-B is present, she should attempt to assess the patient. If the patient refuses transport, you should treat her as any other patient who is refusing care, which includes explaining the consequences of refusal and making a reasonable effort to convince the patient to allow you to transport her. If the patient still refuses, you must obtain a signed release form.

10. B. Opening the airway in infants and small children involves keeping the head in a neutral or *slightly* extended position. Because the occipital region (back of the head) of the skull is proportionately larger in infants and small children when compared to an adult, hyperextension of the neck can result in a reverse flexion of the neck and subsequent airway blockage.

11. D. You should suspect a foreign body airway obstruction in any child who presents with an acute onset of respiratory distress in the absence of fever. If the child is experiencing a mild airway obstruction, in which he or she is moving adequate air, has a normal level of consciousness, and pink skin, do not attempt to relieve the airway obstruction; doing so may result in a severe airway obstruction. Offer oxygen and transport the child to the hospital without delay. If signs of a severe airway obstruction are present (ie, ineffective cough, decreased level of consciousness, cyanosis), you must perform abdominal thrusts until the object is expelled or until the child becomes unconscious.

12. C. Typically, a small child will fear the presence of a stranger in his or her environment and will maintain constant eye contact with the stranger; therefore, inattentiveness to your presence should alert you to the presence of an altered mental status.

13. B. You should never rely on the systolic blood pressure when assessing the perfusion status of anyone. More reliable parameters include assessing peripheral pulses, capillary refill time (most reliable in children younger than 6 years), and the condition and temperature of the skin. Remember that the body's compensatory mechanisms work to maintain the blood pressure, so when it falls, this corresponds to decompensated (late) shock.

14. B. If a child (1 year of age to the onset of puberty [12 to 14 years of age]) with a mild airway obstruction is alert and has adequate air movement (ie, a strong cough, normal skin color), you should offer oxygen, avoid agitating the child, and provide transport to the hospital. Attempts to relieve a mild airway obstruction may result in a severe airway obstruction. If signs of a severe airway obstruction develop, actions to remove the object must be initiated (eg, back blows and chest thrusts in a conscious infant; abdominal thrusts in a conscious adult or child). Finger sweeps are *only* indicated if the patient is unconscious and you can see the object in his or her mouth.

15. C. A heart rate less than 60 beats/min in a child—especially when accompanied by signs of poor perfusion and inadequate breathing—must be managed with chest compressions, ventilation assistance, and rapid transport. Respirations of 8 breaths/min and a heart rate of 50 beats/min will clearly not maintain adequate oxygenation and perfusion in a child.

16. C. Blood loss of up to 500 mL after delivery is considered normal and usually is well tolerated by the mother. However, any bleeding, regardless of the severity, with accompanying signs of shock, must be managed accordingly. In this case, you must apply 100% oxygen, treat the patient for shock by elevating the legs and providing warmth, and provide rapid transport to the hospital while massaging the uterus en route. Dressings should never be packed into the vagina because the bleeding is coming from a source that you cannot control. Additionally, these dressings will then have to be removed at the hospital.

17. B. Care for a prolapsed umbilical cord includes placing your gloved fingers into the vagina and lifting the presenting part of the baby off of the umbilical cord. Continued pressure on the umbilical cord will cut off the baby's oxygen supply. In addition, you should keep the cord moist by covering it in saline-soaked dressings. You should also give the mother 100% oxygen and provide rapid transport to the hospital.

18. A. Initial care for any patient who is seizing—pregnant or otherwise—involves ensuring a patent airway, adequate ventilation, and administering 100% oxygen. If the patient is breathing inadequately, ventilation assistance is indicated. The pregnant patient should be placed on her left side; this will prevent supine hypotensive syndrome—a condition in which the pregnant uterus compresses the inferior vena cava and reduces cardiac output.

19. B. High fever and an alerted mental status indicate sepsis (severe infection). A generalized rash should alert you to the possibility of meningitis—a condition caused by infection and inflammation of the meninges that protect the brain and spinal cord. Children with meningitis are at risk for seizures, usually due to increased intracranial pressure (ICP) and/or high fever; therefore, you must continually monitor the child's condition en route to the hospital and be prepared to treat seizures if they occur.

20. A. Common causes of shock in children include infections, dehydration, and blood loss from trauma. Less common causes include allergic reactions (anaphylaxis) cardiac failure, and poisonings.

21. A. It is relatively common for children to vomit following a head injury such as a concussion. In adults, vomiting—though less common—is an ominous sign and indicates increased intracranial pressure. You must always be prepared for vomiting and have suctioning equipment readily available when managing the patient with a head injury.

22. A. During the initial assessment of a child with trauma, after providing manual stabilization of the head and opening the airway with a jaw-thrust maneuver, you must ensure that the airway is clear. Any fluids in the mouth (eg, blood, vomitus) must be suctioned immediately in order to prevent pulmonary aspiration. Once the airway is clear, this child will require assisted ventilations; slow, irregular respirations will not provide adequate minute volume. Insertion of a nasopharyngeal airway is contraindicated in patients with a head injury.

23. B. When performing 2-rescuer CPR on a child (1 year of age to the onset of puberty [12 to 14 years of age]), the chest should be compressed with one *or* two hands (depending on the size of the child), and a compression to ventilation ratio of 15:2 should be delivered. It is important to compress the chest to an adequate depth—one third to one half the anterior-posterior diameter of the chest. The chest should be allowed to fully recoil in between compressions in order to prevent an increase in intrathoracic pressure and decreased blood return to the heart. If an advanced airway device (ie, ET tube, LMA) is not in place, two rescuers should deliver "cycles" of CPR; the compressor should pause briefly so the ventilator can deliver 2 breaths. A compression to ventilation ratio of 30:2 is indicated for one-rescuer child CPR.

24. A. If the child's condition is stable, the parent should be allowed to hold the child during the examination. This will minimize anxiety in the child and will make the assessment easier for you. In general, you should avoid separating the child and parents unless the child's condition warrants it. When assessing the abdomen of any patient, you should always palpate the painful area last.

25. A. Because infants and small children rely heavily on their diaphragm for breathing (as evidenced by belly breathing), elevating their lower extremities can cause the diaphragm to shift into the thoracic cavity and decrease the effectiveness of breathing. Therefore, in the case of this child, you should lower the lower extremities and reassess.

Subtest 6 Practice Exam: Operations (25 items)

1. C. One of the most important attributes of a safe ambulance driver is the ability to drive with due regard for others. This means that the driver must be aware of others around him or her and to keep their safety in mind. The EMT-B should never assume that all drivers will see or hear the ambulance.

2. A. Actual consent, also referred to as expressed consent, is when the patient asks for your help outright. This may include subtle gestures such as extending the arm to you to allow you to take the blood pressure.

3. D. Although your priority at the scene of a crime is to provide care to the patient, you should attempt to accomplish this by manipulating the scene as little as possible in order to preserve potential evidence. If furniture or other objects do not need to be moved to gain access to the patient, they should be left in place. Conversely, if any obstacles impede your care of the patient, they must be moved as needed.

4. C. Generally, escort vehicles should not be used when responding to an emergency scene. The biggest danger of using an escort occurs at intersections, which is where most ambulance crashes occur. Drivers may yield to the escort vehicle, but may not be prepared for a second vehicle following the escort. The only time that an escort may be required is when you are unfamiliar with the location of the patient and need assistance in getting there. If an escort must be used, you must follow at a safe distance of at least 500'.

5. B. After identifying a patient as an organ donor, your care must be focused on transporting the patient to the hospital as soon as possible and providing aggressive management en route. Your main goal is to provide care in an attempt to save the patient's life. Your secondary goal is to provide the same aggressive care in order to keep the patient viable should his injuries be deemed incompatible with life. If this is the case, his organs can potentially be harvested.

6. C. Early CPR and defibrillation are the most crucial initial treatments to provide to a patient in cardiac arrest. Adequately performed CPR can keep the heart and brain oxygenated, thus increasing the chance of defibrillation success. Ventricular fibrillation (V-Fib) is the most common initial rhythm seen in patients with cardiac arrest and requires prompt defibrillation. Untreated V-Fib will rapidly deteriorate to asystole, the mortality rate from which is very high.

7. C. As an EMT-Basic, your primary responsibility is to yourself. An injured or dead EMT is of no use to a patient. After ensuring the safety of yourself, your crew, and any bystanders, patient care should be initiated.

8. D. As soon as you determine that there are more patients than you and your partner can effectively manage, you must immediately request additional help. Waiting until you are overwhelmed with critically injured patients is not the time to call for help. When in doubt, it is best to call for help. You can always cancel any incoming ambulances if you later determine that they are not needed. After you have called for assistance, you should begin triaging and caring for the patients to the best of your ability.

9. A. At the scene a mass-casualty incident, you will be faced with many challenges, including ensuring your safety, extrication, triage, and patient care. In the midst of all of these activities, however, you must never lose sight of your ultimate goal, which is to transport all patients to the hospital as quickly as possible.

10. C. Immediately upon departing the scene with a patient, you should first apprise the dispatcher that you are en route to the hospital. Never leave the dispatcher in the dark, for it is the dispatcher's job to know what units are available to answer emergency calls. Notifying the receiving facility, contacting medical control, and performing a detailed assessment of your patient all can occur while you are en route to the hospital.

11. B. Once you arrive at the scene of a mass-casualty incident where an incident command system has already been established, you must immediately report to the incident commander. This individual will know where help is needed the most and will be able to direct your actions accordingly.

12. D. During triage, patients with an altered mental status, who are in shock, or who have problems with airway, breathing, or circulation, are potentially salvageable and are given immediate priority. Patients who are pulseless and apneic have low priority in a mass-casualty situation. If you focus your efforts on cardiac arrest patients, who will most likely not survive anyway, patients who could have potentially been saved will die as well. Remember, the goal of triage is to provide the greatest good for the greatest number of patients.

13. A. The role of triage officer should be assumed by the most knowledgeable EMS provider at the scene. Knowledge and experience will enable this person to most effectively manage the triage process. Just because a person has been in the field of EMS for a long period of time does not mean that he or she has been active or has maintained clinical competence.

14. A. The goal of an injury prevention program is just that, prevention. If rescue breathing is needed in a situation, the injury has already occurred. As EMS providers, we are consequence managers. Additionally, we have a responsibility to educate the public on how to avoid injuries in the first place.

15. C. Do not resuscitate orders are particularly challenging for the EMT in the field. When presented with documentation, especially if it does not appear to be valid, in this case, an unsigned document, you must err on the side of patient care and continue resuscitative efforts until medical control orders you to stop.

16. B. The United States Department of Transportation's EMT-Basic National Standard Curriculum requires at least one EMT-Basic in the patient compartment of any ambulance; however, two EMT-Bs are preferred. Although the driver does not have to be an EMT-B, he or she must be able to safely and effectively operate the ambulance. Local laws regarding minimum staffing of an ambulance vary from state to state.

17. A. Many components comprise an EMS quality improvement program, including providing continuing education to all personnel, recognizing those who provide consistently competent patient care, and holding all personnel accountable for adhering to the EMS protocols. The ultimate goal, however, is to provide, as a system, a consistently high standard of care to all patients.

18. C. In caring for any patient, it is important that you keep both the patient and family aware of what you are doing. You should avoid medical vernacular whenever possible because most laypeople will not understand what you are saying. The plain English approach is much more effective. When caring for children specifically, you should inform the parents of the need for ambulance transportation and why, which will provide them with the information necessary to make an informed decision. Asking the parents repeatedly how the child was injured may be construed by some as implying that the child was abused.

19. A. Your partner is clearly having difficulty coming to terms with this call's bad outcome. As her partner, you can be most effective during this time by simply listening and allowing her to voice her feelings. Bad feelings should never be kept bottled up. If your partner is still having difficulties, a formal critical incident stress debriefing (CISD) may be needed.

20. C. Patient care activities, especially when the patient is critical, take priority over the completion of your prehospital care report. Once all patient care activities have been completed, you can sit down and complete the form. This is usually accomplished at the hospital.

21. A. When approaching a residence, findings that would suggest an unsafe scene include, among other things, the sound of breaking glass, screaming and yelling, and an unusual silence. Liquid leaking from a wrecked automobile should be assumed to be gasoline and, therefore, dangerous. Although intimidating in appearance, there is no correlation between a person's size and his or her potential for violence.

22. **C.** General guidelines for safe lifting and moving include keeping the weight as close to your body as possible, keeping your back in a straight, locked-in position, using the muscles of your thighs to lift, and avoiding twisting when moving a patient around a corner. Back injuries are the most common injury sustained by the EMT and can be easily avoided if proper lifting and moving techniques are observed.

23. **D.** When caring for a critically injured patient with multiple injuries, the patient's entire body must be immobilized. This is most quickly and effectively accomplished using a long spine board. Vest-style devices or short spine boards take too long to apply and will not provide full body immobilization. The scoop stretcher is effective for maneuvering patients in narrow spaces but will not allow for full spinal immobilization because of the opening down the center of the device.

24. **D.** Immediately after receiving an order from medical control, you should repeat the order back to medical control word for word. This will ensure that you heard correctly and understand the order to be carried out. If you receive an order that seems inappropriate, you should ask the physician to repeat the order back to you for clarification.

25. **C.** The appropriate method for disposing of soiled clothing or any other "nonsharp" contaminated item is to place it in a red biohazard bag. The insignia as well as the red color alerts others that the items within the bag are contaminated.

Practice Final Examination (150 Items)

1. **C.** Snoring respirations, which most commonly result from partial airway obstruction by the tongue, are most rapidly managed by correctly positioning the head. This involves using either the head tilt-chin lift or the jaw-thrust maneuver if trauma is suspected. To further ensure airway patency, an adjunct may need to be inserted.

2. **A.** A rapid trauma assessment would be indicated for any patient with abnormal findings in the initial assessment or when the mechanism of injury warrants it. Significant mechanisms of injury include, among others, falls in the adult of greater than 15′ (or three times the patient's height), penetrating injuries to the head, neck, chest, or abdomen, and multiple long bone fractures.

3. **B.** Recalling the body in the anatomic position, the radius is the lateral bone of the forearm and the ulna is the medial bone. The humerus is the long bone of the upper arm and the clavicle is the collarbone, which extends from the sternum laterally to the shoulder.

4. **C.** When the body attempts to compensate for shock, peripheral vasoconstriction shunts blood away from the skin to the more vital organs in the body such as the brain, heart, lungs, and kidneys. When there is minimal or no peripheral blood flow, the skin assumes a pale appearance.

5. **A.** Pain in the right upper quadrant and skin with a yellowish tinge to it (jaundice) indicates a problem with the liver. Jaundice is the result of an increased production of bilirubin in the liver. Dysfunction of the pancreas would result in possible fluctuations in the levels of blood glucose. Gallbladder inflammation (cholecystitis) typically produces right upper quadrant pain and/or referred pain to the right shoulder that occurs shortly after eating. Dysfunction of the spleen would cause left upper quadrant pain and/or referred pain to the left shoulder.

6. D. Abandonment occurs any time you disengage from a patient while he or she still requires care or you relinquish your responsibility of patient care to a provider of lesser training. If a first responder assumes patient care from an EMT-Intermediate—clearly a provider with a higher level of training—then the EMT-Intermediate has abandoned his or her patient.

7. D. According to the American Heart Association, you should assess the brachial pulse in infants younger than 1 year of age. The carotid or femoral pulse can be assessed in children older than 1 year of age. A carotid pulse is difficult to locate in infants because they have minimal space between their head and shoulders.

8. A. Any trauma patient with maxillofacial trauma is at an extremely high risk of airway compromise. The airway can be compromised by either mandibular fractures, in which the tongue may occlude the airway, or severe oral bleeding, in which blood clots can obstruct the airway.

9. B. The patient's airway must be clear of foreign bodies or secretions before it can be managed. If the patient begins to vomit, he must first be rolled onto his side to allow for drainage of the vomitus and then provided suction. If the patient is injured, this must be accomplished carefully, without manipulating the spine. After the airway is clear, it should be managed accordingly.

10. B. The components of the scene size-up include determining scene safety, assessing the mechanism of injury or nature of illness, noting the number of patients, and determining if additional help is needed. Personal protective equipment should be donned prior to beginning the scene size-up.

11. D. The oropharyngeal airway is used to keep the tongue off of the posterior pharynx and is indicated for unconscious patients without a gag reflex.

12. D. Only one critical patient per ambulance can be managed effectively with two EMTs. As soon as you determine that the critical patient count exceeds your capabilities, you should immediately call for additional help.

13. D. Even though this patient has chest pain and prescribed nitroglycerin, you must first complete a focused history and physical examination and obtain baseline vital signs. Medical control will need this information—specifically the patient's blood pressure—in order to determine whether you should assist the patient with his nitroglycerin.

14. D. The gallbladder, which concentrates and stores bile, is not an endocrine organ. Endocrine organs produce hormones, which regulate other body organs and systems. The thyroid regulates metabolism, the pancreas produces insulin and glucagon, and the pituitary, which is located within the brain, is the "master" endocrine gland and regulates the function of all endocrine glands in the body.

15. B. Any injury that jeopardizes the airway has priority over all else. If bleeding within the mouth is not suctioned immediately, blood will be aspirated in the lungs, and the patient will become more hypoxic.

16. A. In the absence of any witnesses, any patient found unconscious should be assumed to be a trauma patient until proven otherwise. Appropriate measures such as spinal immobilization must be taken.

17. A. The detailed physical examination usually is performed on a critically injured patient or an unresponsive medical patient. Whether the patient you are caring for is injured or is ill, the detailed examination should be performed in the back of the ambulance while you are en route to the hospital. The purpose of the detailed physical examination is to detect and treat less obvious injuries or illnesses, some of which may be life threatening.

18. C. Flushed or red skin commonly is seen in patients who are exposed to heat. Fever also can cause flushed skin. Shock and low blood pressure generally cause the skin to become pale, and hypoxia causes cyanosis, a bluish-gray tint to the skin.

19. C. As soon as an open pneumothorax is discovered, you must take immediate steps to prevent air from entering the wound or further hypoxia will occur. This is most effectively accomplished by placing an occlusive dressing over the wound and securing it on three sides. A porous dressing will not effectively seal the wound. The patient must then be monitored for signs of a developing tension pneumothorax, such as worsening shortness of breath, cyanosis, or shock. If a tension pneumothorax develops, the unsecured end of the dressing must be lifted to allow the buildup of air in the pleural space to escape.

20. B. Wheezing, hives, and edema are hallmark findings of an allergic reaction. In this case, the patient is having a severe reaction. Although wheezing is a classic finding in patients with asthma, hives and facial edema are not associated with asthma. Wheezing typically does not occur with heat-related problems. Unless a poisonous plant is ingested, it is likely that exposure to a poisonous plant will result in local irritation.

21. B. Because nitroglycerin dilates the blood vessels, including those within the brain, the brain is engorged with blood, which typically gives the patient a pounding headache. This is a usual and expected side effect of the drug.

22. C. Once cardiac arrest is confirmed, the highest priority is to attach the AED to determine if the patient has a shockable rhythm. While your partner gets the AED from the ambulance, you should begin CPR. Once the AED is available, it should immediately be attached and the patient defibrillated if indicated.

23. C. Prescribed inhalers, such as albuterol (Ventolin) and isoetharene (Bronkosol), are in a class of drugs referred to as bronchodilators. They relax the smooth muscle found within the bronchioles in the lungs, which causes them to dilate. This effect improves air passage and enhances the patient's ability to breathe.

24. C. Signs and symptoms that suggest cardiac compromise include, among others, chest pain or pressure, dyspnea, anxiety, and diaphoresis. Headache is not a common presenting symptom associated with cardiac compromise.

25. B. The single most important parameter to monitor in a patient with suspected head trauma is level of consciousness. It should be monitored frequently in order to determine whether the patient's condition is improving (ie, concussion), or worsening (ie, intracerebral hemorrhage). In general, level of consciousness also serves as the most reliable indicator of perfusion.

26. B. The mid-upper region of the abdomen is referred to as the epigastrium because of its location over the stomach (epi = upon, gastric = stomach). This is a common site of pain or discomfort in cardiac patients, which frequently causes them to attribute the pain to indigestion.

27. C. During anaphylaxis, the histamines released from the immune system cause two deleterious effects that result in shock (hypoperfusion): vasodilation, which causes the blood pressure to fall and bronchoconstriction, which impairs breathing.

28. D. In the patient with diabetes, hypoglycemia is called insulin shock and presents with cool, clammy skin and a rapid onset. The brain is critically dependent on glucose and responds quickly when the body is in short supply. Hyperglycemia or diabetic coma typically presents with warm, dry skin and a slow onset, sometimes occurring over a period of days.

29. A. Bradycardia is not commonly associated with either hyperglycemia or hypoglycemia. Tachycardia and combativeness can occur in patients with hyperglycemia or hypoglycemia. A fruity breath odor is noted exclusively in patients with diabetic ketoacidosis (diabetic coma).

30. B. Any patient with a significant, most often negative, life change is at risk for suicide. Common catalysts to suicide include the loss of a loved one or a job, financial difficulties, and the diagnosis of a terminal disease.

31. A. You should first assess the rate, regularity, depth, and quality of the patient's respirations. All of this information is necessary so that you can provide the most appropriate airway management. You should not rely on respiratory rate alone to guide your management. A patient can be breathing rapidly or slowly, yet effectively.

32. D. Tidal volume is the amount of air, in milliliters, breathed into the lungs in a single breath. The most effective way to assess tidal volume is to evaluate the rise of the patient's chest. A reduced tidal volume is manifested as shallow respirations, which most likely will necessitate assisted ventilations.

33. C. In the field, a do-not-resuscitate order must be validated by a physician. You must not withhold resuscitative efforts while awaiting this validation. CPR must be continued until medical control is contacted and orders you to stop. When in doubt, resuscitate.

34. B. When assessing the abdomen of a child or adult, you should determine the location of the pain and palpate that area last. Begin by palpating the abdomen furthest away from the area of pain; in this case, the left upper quadrant is furthest away from the right lower quadrant. Palpating the painful area first will interfere with the rest of your assessment because the patient will be in significant pain and will likely not remain still during the remainder of the assessment. This is especially true in children. Auscultation of bowel sounds is generally not performed in the prehospital setting; little, if any, information will be gained from doing so.

35. A. Although each state may have slightly differing reporting laws, most require the EMT-B to report cases such as child or elderly abuse, sexual assault, animal bites, and injury that occurs during the commission of a felony. Injury to a minor is typically not a reportable case unless abuse is suspected. Motor vehicle crashes and drug overdoses are not reportable cases either unless they occur during the commission of a felony.

36. C. The set of legal regulations and ethical considerations that define the job of the EMT-B is called the scope of practice. The scope of practice provides a clear delineation of the EMT-B's roles and responsibilities. Duty to act is defined as a legal obligation to respond to every call for help while on duty and in your jurisdiction, whether you are paid for your services or not. Confidentiality entails not releasing any patient information to those not directly involved in the care of the patient. The Medical Practices Act describes the minimum qualifications of those who may engage in emergency medical care and establishes a means of certification.

37. C. Abdominal trauma commonly occurs in children as the result of motor vehicle versus pedestrian accidents. The contusions over the left upper quadrant and the signs of shock suggest significant injury to the spleen.

38. C. The AED is only applied to patients in cardiac arrest (eg, pulseless and apneic), whether the arrest was witnessed or unwitnessed. According to the 2005 Emergency Cardiac Care (ECC) guidelines, AEDs can safely be used in children between 1 and 8 years of age in conjunction with a dose-attenuating system (energy reducer) and pediatric pads. However, if pediatric pads and an energy reducer are unavailable, a regular AED should be used. A nitroglycerin patch is not a contraindication to the use of an AED; simply remove the patch (with gloved hands) and apply the AED as usual.

39. A. Nighttime traffic crashes, especially those that occur on a highway, pose a significant risk to the safety of the EMT. Therefore, immediately upon exiting the ambulance, the concern for oncoming traffic should be at the front of the EMT's mind. Often, other drivers can be blinded by all of the emergency lighting and inadvertently veer off of the road and strike the rescuer.

40. A. Components of the initial assessment for both conscious and unconscious patients include assessing and managing the airway and assessing and managing circulation, which includes controlling any major bleeding; assessing the rate, regularity, and quality of the pulse; and assessing the color, condition, and temperature of the skin.

41. D. Upon arrival at the scene where CPR is in progress, you must first conduct an initial assessment to confirm that the patient is indeed pulseless and apneic. Often, bystanders who are not properly trained in assessing for a carotid pulse will begin CPR when the patient really does not need it.

42. C. Most adult out-of-hospital cardiac arrests are the result of a cardiac arrhythmia, most commonly ventricular fibrillation. This finding underscores the importance of early defibrillation immediately upon confirmation of cardiac arrest in the adult.

43. B. As previously mentioned, ventricular fibrillation is the most common initial presenting cardiac arrhythmia in adult cardiac arrest patients. Ventricular fibrillation is a quivering of the heart muscle that does not produce a palpable pulse and is due to chaotic electrical discharge of the cardiac cells. The most effective therapy for this deadly rhythm is defibrillation.

44. D. As soon as the newborn's head has delivered, you should first suction the mouth, then the nose. As the infant is forced through the birth canal, the thoracic cavity is squeezed, which causes the infant to expel amniotic fluid from the lungs. If this fluid is not thoroughly suctioned, it can be aspirated, resulting in hypoxia and a difficult resuscitation.

45. D. Central cyanosis (cyanosis to the head, face, and trunk) alone initially should be treated with blow-by oxygen; however, when it is accompanied by a heart rate that is less than 100 beats/min, artificial ventilations should be initiated and continued until the heart rate exceeds 100 beats/min. Newborn bradycardia is defined as a heart rate of less than 100 beats/min.

46. A. Battery is defined as unlawfully touching another person without his or her consent. Obtaining consent from every conscious and alert patient prior to rendering care is of paramount importance.

47. A. Effective chest compressions are essential for providing blood flow during CPR. To perform "effective" chest compressions, the EMT should "push hard and push fast." Compress the adult's chest at a rate of 100 compressions/min to a depth of 1 ½" to 2". Allow the chest to *completely* recoil after each compression, and allow equal time for compression and relaxation. Minimize interruptions in CPR to 10 seconds or less. Obviously, chest compressions must be paused when using the AED to analyze the patient's cardiac rhythm or defibrillating and when assessing for a pulse.

48. D. The most common cause of cardiac arrest in infants and children is failure of the respiratory system. Their hearts generally are healthy, and they rarely go into ventricular fibrillation. Aggressive and effective airway management is essential in the prevention of pediatric cardiac arrest.

49. A. Fibrinolytic (clot-buster) therapy is critical to a patient who is having a stroke if it is initiated within 3 hours after the onset of symptoms. In addition to providing 100% oxygen, it is extremely important that you provide rapid transport to the hospital for this therapy. Because fibrinolytic therapy decreases the blood's ability to clot, its use should be limited to patients with ischemic strokes. It would increase intracerebral bleeding in patients with hemorrhagic stroke; therefore, fibrinolytic therapy should not be provided to these patients.

50. A. Indications for oral glucose include patients with known diabetes who are suspected of having hypoglycemia (insulin shock). The patient must be conscious and alert enough to be able to swallow the glucose, which comes in a tube of gel. If the patient is unconscious or otherwise unable to swallow the glucose, you should provide rapid transport, providing the appropriate airway management, and consider an ALS rendezvous.

51. C. There are two indications for removing an impaled object: when the object is causing airway compromise and when the object interferes with your ability to perform CPR. A knife impaled in the center of the chest in a patient who is in cardiac arrest must be carefully removed, and bleeding should be controlled, an occlusive dressing applied if needed, and CPR initiated.

52. B. Nitroglycerin is contraindicated in patients who do not have a prescription for nitroglycerin, in those with a systolic BP less than 100 mm Hg, and in patients who have taken medications for erectile dysfunction (ED)—especially within the previous 24 hours. Such medications include sildenafil (Viagra), vardenafil (Levitra) and tadalafil (Cialis). Because ED drugs and nitroglycerin both cause vasodilation, concomitant use of these drugs may result in life-threatening hypotension.

53. D. Because of the signs and symptoms that this patient is exhibiting, you must be immediately concerned with the potential for closure of the airway and be prepared to assist ventilations. Signs of airway burns include respiratory distress, singed nasal hairs, a brassy cough, difficulty breathing, and coughing up sooty sputum. Infection, the burns themselves, and hypothermia should concern you; however, airway problems clearly pose the greatest life threats.

54. C. You must first address problems that pose the greatest threat to life. The injury to the groin area most likely is an arterial bleed from the femoral artery, and immediate direct pressure must be applied to the groin area. Because the patient is screaming in pain, it is clear that his airway is patent. After the bleeding has been controlled, 100% oxygen should be administered and shock measures initiated while the patient is rapidly transported to the hospital.

55. C. Closed head injuries can cause a variety of signs and symptoms. In addition to pupillary changes (typically unequal pupils), a classic finding that indicates increased intracranial pressure is called "Cushing's triad," which is a trio of findings, including hypertension, bradycardia, and altered respirations, which can vary from slow and irregular to rapid and deep.

56. C. Tidal volume is the amount of air, in milliliters, that is breathed into the lungs in a single breath. Shallow respirations (minimal chest rise) would indicate that the mechanics of breathing are not sufficient enough to bring adequate volumes of air into the lungs. Patients with shallow breathing typically require positive pressure ventilation in order to increase tidal volume and enhance oxygenation.

57. B. After attaching the nonrebreathing mask to the oxygen source, the flowmeter must be set at 15 L/min. The reservoir bag is then prefilled with oxygen, which will allow the delivery of up to 100% oxygen to the patient.

58. B. Because this patient is only able to speak in minimal word sentences (two-word dyspnea), she is exhibiting signs of inadequate breathing and must have assisted ventilations. If her breathing continues as it is, she will become extremely hypoxic and may lose consciousness. Because this patient is conscious, you must explain to her that every time she takes in a breath, the bag-valve-mask device will be squeezed so that adequate volume can be delivered. Clearly, this can cause the patient great anxiety, so your reassurance during this procedure is important.

59. A. The goal of providing artificial ventilation is to provide adequate tidal volume to the patient so that enough oxygen is delivered to the cells of the body. The most effective way to determine if adequate tidal volume is being delivered is to watch for the chest to rise during each ventilation. Other signs of adequate artificial ventilation include improvement in skin color, the return of the heart rate to a normal range, and ensuring that you are ventilating the patient at the appropriate rate (10 to 12 breaths/min in the apneic adult with a pulse; 8 to 10 breaths/min in the pulseless and apneic adult).

60. A. Before assisting a patient with any medication other than oxygen, the EMT-B must obtain permission from medical control. In this case, the physician probably will allow you to help the patient take one more puff from the patient's inhaler. Generally, up to three puffs from an inhaler are delivered in the field. It is important for you to ask the patient how many puffs were taken from the inhaler before you arrived.

61. A. Signs of a narcotic overdose from drugs such as heroin, morphine, Meperidine (Demerol), or codeine include altered mental status, slow, shallow breathing, and pupillary constriction. Narcotics are central nervous system depressants that, when taken in excess, suppress the vital functions necessary for life, such as breathing, heart rate, and blood pressure. Barbiturates produce the same effects; however, the pupils are typically dilated, not constricted. Marijuana and amphetamine drugs are central nervous system stimulants and would thus cause the patient to become restless or even combative.

62. B. When managing any patient with an emotional or psychiatric problem, your primary concern is your own safety. Safely transporting the patient to the hospital is your ultimate goal. If possible, you should attempt to obtain a medical history and should take any of the patient's prescribed medications to the hospital. However, this should not supercede your own safety or interfere with safely transporting the patient.

63. C. As soon as you determine that an adult patient is apneic, your first action is to deliver two rescue breaths (1 second per breath; enough to produce visible chest rise) and then assess for a carotid pulse. If a pulse is present, an airway adjunct should be inserted and rescue breathing continued (10 to 12 breaths/min) with close monitoring of the pulse. If the patient is pulseless, CPR should be initiated and the cardiac rhythm analyzed with an AED as soon as possible.

64. C. First, you must determine the child's weight in kilograms (kg). Either of the following formulae can be used to determine a patient's weight in kilograms:

Formula 1: weight (in pounds) ÷ 2.2 = weight in kg

Formula 2: weight (in pounds) ÷ 2 − 10% = weight in kg

On the basis of the above formulae, a 40-pound child weighs 18 kg. Using formula 1, the equation is as follows: 40 (weight in pounds) ÷ 2.2 = 18.18 (18 [rounded to the nearest tenth]). Using formula 2, the equation is as follows: 40 (weight in pounds) ÷ 2 = 20 − 10% (2) = 18. Since the drug order is for 1 g/kg, you should administer 18 g of activated charcoal to your 40-pound patient.

65. C. If you can see the umbilical cord wrapped around the newborn's neck (nuchal cord) when the head delivers, you should gently attempt to slide the cord from around the neck. If this is unsuccessful, you should clamp and cut the cord and continue the delivery. You must never pull on the umbilical cord. In cases where the umbilical cord is prolapsed (the cord presents before the baby), it should be kept moist and the patient rapidly transported.

66. B. As evidenced by her recent illness and fever (102.5°F), this child has likely experienced a febrile seizure. Appropriate treatment for the child following a febrile seizure involves ensuring a patent airway, administering oxygen (the blow-by technique is generally better tolerated than a mask), removing the child's clothing, applying towels moistened with tepid water to slowly lower the body temperature, and transporting to the hospital. Since the child is no longer seizing, anticonvulsant drugs are not indicated. Do not rapidly cool the child with cold water; doing so may cause the child to shiver—a mechanism that produces body heat—which may cause an abrupt rise in body temperature and another seizure.

67. D. A universal compression to ventilation ratio of 30:2 is used for all one-rescuer CPR (adult, child, and infant), with the exception of the newborn. A compression to ventilation ratio of 3:1 is used for newborns (one- and two-rescuer). Two-rescuer infant and child CPR is performed at a compression to ventilation ratio of 15:2.

68. B. After the AED delivers a shock, you should immediately begin or resume CPR. Perform 5 cycles (about 2 minutes) of CPR and then reanalyze the child's cardiac rhythm. If the AED states that a shock is advised, defibrillate without delay. If the AED states "no shock advised", assess for a pulse. If a pulse is present, reassess airway and breathing and treat accordingly. If the pulse is absent, resume CPR and reanalyze the cardiac rhythm in 2 minutes. Interruptions in CPR should be minimal (10 seconds or less).

69. B. After an advanced airway device has been placed (ie, ET tube, LMA), you should ventilate the child (and adult) in cardiac arrest at a rate of 8 to 10 breaths/min. Healthcare providers often deliver excessive ventilation—particularly when an advanced airway device is in place. Excessive ventilation (eg, hyperventilation) is detrimental because it impedes blood flow back to the heart, thereby decreasing coronary and cerebral blood flow due to increased intrathoracic pressure. Hyperventilation also increases the risk of regurgitation and aspiration.

70. B. Gastric distention can be lethal if not caught and managed appropriately in children. As air insufflates the stomach, the diaphragm is pushed into the thoracic cavity, which decreases the amount of air that can fill the lungs. This results in decreased ventilatory volumes during artificial ventilation. Respiratory failure is the most common cause of cardiac arrest in children.

71. B. In children younger than 6 years, capillary refill serves as an excellent indicator of perfusion by indicating oxygen delivery to the capillaries. It is important to remember that factors such as cold temperature affect capillary refill. Early in shock (hypoperfusion), the heart rate increases, as does the respiratory rate in an attempt to compensate for decreases in oxygen. When these compensatory mechanisms fail, the blood pressure falls, which makes blood pressure a very unreliable indicator of perfusion.

72. C. Some adults cannot tolerate the oppressive feeling of an oxygen mask over their face, although children are more commonly less tolerant than adults. You should provide reassurance to the patient and apply a nasal cannula at 2 to 6 L/min, which will likely be better tolerated.

73. D. Signs of inadequate breathing in both conscious and unconscious patients include a respiratory rate that is too fast or too slow; shallow, irregular, or gasping respirations; and respiratory noises such as wheezing, stridor, or gurgling.

74. C. During initial attempts at providing artificial ventilation, the pocket mask with supplemental oxygen and one-way valve should be used. As opposed to the one-person bag-valve-mask technique, the pocket mask is easier for one person to operate and can deliver greater tidal volumes. In addition, a better sense of ventilatory compliance can be felt by the rescuer when using the pocket mask. The most common problem associated with the one-person BVM technique is difficulty in maintaining an effective mask-to-face seal.

75. A. According to the Centers for Disease Control and Prevention, the most effective way to prevent the spread of disease is to frequently and effectively wash your hands. Remaining up to date with your immunizations, the regular use of gloves with all patients, and wearing a mask when managing a patient with a communicable disease such as tuberculosis will decrease your chance of disease exposure.

76. A. If you discover that you forgot to write pertinent information on your prehospital care report after leaving a copy at the hospital, your most appropriate action would be to write the information on an addendum and attach it to the original care report. A copy of the addendum also should be sent to the receiving facility. Once you leave a copy of your prehospital care report at the hospital, you must not add anything to the original. Legally, this would result in two different records for the same patient.

77. B. Just because the patient is 92 years old does not mean that she can no longer make an informed decision. In cases where any patient refuses care, after determining that the patient is of sound mind and body, you must inform the patient of the risks of refusing care, namely death. If the patient is aware of and willing to accept those consequences, a signed refusal must be obtained from the patient.

78. D. One of the most effective ways to reduce stress in a bystander at the scene of a mass-casualty incident is to assign the bystander a task that is not related to patient care. This may involve assisting other bystanders who are having difficulties as well or providing water to the rescuers. An obviously distressed bystander should not simply be sent away from the scene, but should be looked at as a patient as well.

79. D. A patient may be treated under the law of implied consent any time he or she is unconscious or considered not to be of sound mind and body to the extent that he or she can make an informed decision. Examples of such patients include those who are intoxicated or who otherwise have an altered mental status (ie, stroke or hypoglycemia). Patients younger than 18 years may also be treated using implied consent, unless the patient is female and is emancipated or pregnant.

80. A. Chest pain, pressure, or discomfort (usually lasting > 15 minutes) is present in the majority of patients experiencing acute myocardial infarction (AMI). Other common signs and symptoms include shortness of breath, nausea, and diaphoresis. However, elderly female patients—especially those with diabetes—are more likely to present with atypical or unusual signs and symptoms than any other patient population. Diabetic neuropathy—a condition associated with diabetes—results in decreased sensitivity to pain; therefore, the patient may present without any pain or discomfort. Sometimes, the only presenting signs or symptoms of AMI are generalized weakness, fatigue, or other nonspecific findings.

81. D. An irregular pulse indicates abnormalities in the electrical conduction system of the heart. The electrical conduction system, beginning with the sinoatrial node as the primary pacemaker, is responsible for initiating the electrical impulses that stimulate the myocardium to contract. An irregular pulse could indicate potentially lethal arrhythmias that could result in cardiac arrest. You must document an irregular pulse and pass this important finding to the emergency department.

82. B. The patient is conscious, alert, and talking clearly, which indicates that he has a patent airway. If the arterial bleeding is not controlled immediately, the patient will bleed to death; therefore, you should control bleeding first. Immediately after controlling the bleeding, you should apply oxygen.

83. C. No airway, no patient! If your initial attempt to ventilate the patient is unsuccessful, you should reposition the head and reattempt to ventilate. If you are still unsuccessful, you must begin airway obstruction removal techniques and transport immediately. In unconscious patients with a severe airway obstruction (adult, child, and infant), perform chest compressions, visualize the airway for the obstruction (remove it *only* if you see it; no blind finger sweeps), and attempt to ventilate. Repeat this cycle of events until the obstruction is relieved or advanced life support personnel assume care of the patient.

84. B. Using the adult Rule of Nines, the head accounts for 9% of the body surface area (BSA), the anterior chest for 9% (the entire anterior trunk accounts for 18%), and the anterior upper extremities for 4.5% each (each entire arm is 9% of the BSA). On the basis of this, the patient has sustained 27% full-thickness burns.

85. D. The "R" in OPQRST stands for radiation. An appropriate way to determine whether the pain radiates or not is to ask the patient if the pain remains in one place or if it moves around. If you use the term "radiating pain," chances are the patient will not understand what you are asking.

86. A. The correct method of inserting a nasopharyngeal airway is to lubricate the device with a water-soluble gel and insert the airway with the bevel facing the septum or the base of the nostril. If resistance is met, you should attempt to insert the airway into the other nostril. Forcing the airway into place will cause trauma to the nasal mucosa and unnecessary bleeding, which the patient could potentially aspirate.

87. A. Cardiac output is the amount of blood ejected from the ventricles in a single minute. To best obtain an indication of cardiac output, you should assess the rate and quality of the pulse. A rapid, bounding pulse indicates increased cardiac output during the compensation phase in patients with shock. As the pulse quality becomes weak or "thready," the cardiac output has fallen significantly, which corresponds with a falling blood pressure.

88. C. After any device is used that has the potential for causing an accidental needle stick or is otherwise contaminated, it should be placed in a puncture-proof container, which usually is red and has a biohazard logo on it. The cover of the auto-injector should never be replaced, nor should a needle be recapped.

89. C. Once an ingested poison gets into the system, it can affect multiple organ systems. Signs that this is occurring include tachycardia and hypotension. Other signs might include weakness or an altered level of consciousness. Local effects of an ingested poison include nausea and vomiting as the poison irritates the gastric lining, and burns in and around the mouth.

90. A. General rules to follow when attempting to rescue a patient from the water include "throw, tow, row, and then go." In this case, the swimmer should be thrown a rope or flotation device to grab on to. Going into the water to retrieve the swimmer should be a last resort. The rescuer who jumps into the water must be a strong swimmer because patients who are in danger of drowning are panicked and will make every attempt to keep themselves afloat, even if it means forcing the rescuer underwater.

91. A. In cases where a patient is breathing inadequately or not at all and is regurgitating secretions at the same time, you must address both issues. This is accomplished most effectively by suctioning for 15 seconds and then ventilating for 2 minutes. This alternating sequence should be repeated until all secretions are cleared from the airway.

92. C. After establishing the patient's level of consciousness, you must next make sure that he or she is breathing adequately and initiate the most appropriate airway management. Management will involve using either supplemental oxygen or positive pressure ventilations. Determining the cause of a patient's altered mental status is an important aspect of the assessment, but it should not precede ensuring effective breathing and circulation. Patients with altered mental status or those who cannot swallow should not be given anything by mouth because it may be aspirated into their lungs.

93. A. All patients with severe pain, including those with severe abdominal pain, require immediate transport, and 100% oxygen is clearly indicated. Most patients with severe abdominal pain will prefer to lie on their side with their knees drawn up into their chest. This takes pressure off of the large abdominal muscle mass and often affords them some relief. The patient should not be given anything to drink because surgery may be required. Auscultating for bowel sounds is not considered a useful sign and will provide you with little or no information. The goal is to transport the patient to the hospital where definitive care can be provided.

94. B. After a generalized (grand mal) motor seizure, the patient typically will be confused, sleepy, or in some cases, combative. This is referred to as the postictal phase of the seizure. Eventually, the patient's level of consciousness will improve.

95. B. You must deliver adequate tidal volume to the patient to cause sufficient chest rise. If initial ventilations cause minimal rise of the patient's chest, you may need to increase the volume of ventilations by squeezing the bag harder until the chest rises adequately. If this is ineffective, you may need to reevaluate the size of the mask that you are using or clear the patient's airway of any secretions.

96. D. Because of the significant mechanism of injury (a fall of greater than 15'), spinal injury must be assumed. The fact that the patient is unconscious reinforces the assumption that he sustained significant injury. The first step in managing this patient is to manually stabilize his head and perform a jaw-thrust maneuver, both of which can be accomplished simultaneously. After the head has been stabilized and the airway opened, you can proceed with assessing the respirations.

97. D. Shallow respirations, regardless of the respiratory rate, are not sufficient to provide adequate tidal volume for oxygenation. Some form of positive pressure ventilation (ie, BVM device or pocket mask) must be initiated. Although the patient is conscious, if no measures are taken to improve the tidal volume, he will become more hypoxic and eventually lose consciousness and become apneic.

98. C. Signs of inadequate artificial ventilation include an uneven (asymmetrical) rise of the chest, minimal chest rise, an abnormal heart rate, continued cyanosis, and a rate of artificial ventilation that is too fast or too slow.

99. B. Prior to delivering a shock with the AED, the EMT must verbally and visually ensure that nobody is touching the patient. After this has been accomplished, deliver the shock without delay and then immediately begin or resume CPR. AEDs have a high specificity for recognizing shockable cardiac rhythms; therefore, reanalyzing the patient's cardiac rhythm to confirm that a shock is indicated will only waste time in delivering the shock.

100. A. Management of a patient with full-thickness burns includes applying 100% oxygen; dry, sterile dressings; warmth to the patient; and providing rapid transport. Moist, sterile dressings should not be applied to full-thickness burns because the risk of inducing hypothermia and infection is increased.

101. C. To ensure delivery of as close to 100% oxygen as possible, you must first set the flowmeter to 15 L/min and then preinflate the reservoir bag on a nonrebreathing mask before applying the mask to the patient. When the patient inhales, 100% oxygen is inspired directly from this bag. The one-way valves on the side of the mask close during inspiration, allowing no outside carbon dioxide to mix with the oxygen from the reservoir. Following preinflation, you must make sure that the mask is secured to the patient's face.

102. D. Because of the absence of trauma, the patient's airway should be opened with a head tilt-chin lift maneuver. To further ensure airway patency, a nasopharyngeal airway must be inserted. Because the patient is semiconscious, she will likely not tolerate an oropharyngeal airway. Remember, you must first open the patient's airway and secure it with an adjunct if needed prior to assessing respiratory effort.

103. B. Shallow respirations (reduced tidal volume) at a rate of 26 breaths/min will not provide adequate minute volume. Therefore, you must initiate positive pressure ventilations with 100% oxygen using either a pocket mask or a bag-valve-mask device. Passive oxygenation devices (eg, nonrebreathing mask, simple face mask) will be of little benefit to a patient with inadequate breathing.

104. A. A patient who has shallow respirations is not inhaling sufficient volumes of air into the lungs so that the blood can be oxygenated effectively. Tidal volume is the amount of air breathed into the lungs in a single breath; therefore, shallow breathing will result in a decreased tidal volume. These patients need some form of positive pressure ventilation.

105. C. Cyanosis, a bluish-gray tint to the skin, is a reflection of inadequate amounts of oxygen in the arterial blood. More specifically, cyanosis indicates that a significant amount of hemoglobin has dissociated from the red blood cell and the arterial blood is less able to carry oxygen. Patients with cyanosis must be evaluated further so that the underlying cause can be determined and managed appropriately.

106. B. The mechanism of injury for this patient was significant. After taking the appropriate BSI precautions, you must first manually stabilize the patient's head. Then, the patient must be log rolled as a unit into a supine position where you can gain access to his airway.

107. B. Because of the significant mechanism of injury, after the initial assessment and appropriate management have been completed, you must next perform a rapid trauma assessment to look for and treat other life threats. Vital signs are typically obtained at the end of the rapid trauma assessment, and the detailed physical exam for a critically injured patient should occur in the back of the ambulance while en route to the hospital. Critically injured patients must be immobilized to a long spine board. The vest-style device takes too long to apply.

108. C. The consequences of refusal should be explained to any patient who refuses EMS treatment and/or transport. After establishing that the patient is in a position to be able to refuse treatment and transport (ie, she is of legal age and sound mind and body), you must advise her that because of the significant mechanism of injury, the potential for critical injury exists for her as well, even though she may feel fine now. Once this is explained, and the patient understands the consequences, a signed refusal must be obtained from the patient.

109. D. Any time a patient's condition deteriorates—such as your patient whose respirations have increased—you should immediately repeat the initial assessment and adjust your treatment accordingly. After stabilizing the patient's condition, you should reassess vital signs—including oxygen saturation—and then notify the receiving facility.

110. B. The most reliable indicator of an underlying injury is the presence of palpable pain, specifically point tenderness at the site of the injury. This applies not only to spinal injury, but any potential underlying injury.

111. A. A 3-year-old child typically is very attentive to his or her surroundings, especially when a stranger enters the environment. The fact that this child does not acknowledge your presence is an abnormal sign and indicates that the child is hypoxic. This child must therefore be managed aggressively to prevent respiratory arrest and subsequent cardiac arrest.

112. C. Most children with febrile seizures do not have any permanent aftereffects. The most appropriate management is to offer the child oxygen, allow a parent to accompany and hold the child, and provide transport to the hospital in the ambulance. Although most seizures in children result from a simple infection that causes an abrupt rise in body temperature, other illnesses such as meningitis and encephalitis can cause seizures as well and are far more serious. For this reason, any child with fever and seizures must be evaluated in the emergency department. Rapid cooling of the child in cold water is likely to result in shivering, which could abruptly increase the child's temperature and cause another seizure. Children with a fever should be kept cool during transport, but not to a point where they shiver.

113. C. EMT-Bs always must keep the possibility of child abuse in the back of their minds when dealing with an injured child. Signs that would indicate abuse include, but are not limited to, bruises in areas that are not likely to be injured, such as the thigh, back, and chest; multiple bruises in varying colors, indicating various stages of healing; conflicting stories among caregivers; injuries that are beyond the developmental abilities of the child, such as a 1-year-old child who has "fallen from her bicycle"; and cases in which the child does not look at the parents or cling to them as one would expect an injured child to do. Siblings of an abused child are typically not curious onlookers as they have become accustomed to the abusive environment. As an EMT-B, you have a legal obligation to report any and all cases of suspected child abuse to the emergency department physician. Never accuse anyone of abusing a child. If you are wrong, you could be held liable for slander.

114. B. An ectopic pregnancy must be assumed, until proven otherwise, in any woman of childbearing age who has abdominal pain. Because her last menstrual period occurred 2 months earlier and she has pain and vaginal bleeding, this patient is a "textbook" candidate for an ectopic pregnancy.

115. C. The source of bleeding from the vagina cannot be directly controlled in the field. You should never pack or place any dressings directly into the vagina because they will only have to be removed at the hospital. Instead, you should place a trauma dressing or similar material over the vagina, treat the patient for shock, and provide prompt transport to the hospital.

116. D. Children with no fever who have a sudden onset of respiratory distress should be managed for a foreign body airway obstruction. Infections such as epiglottitis also cause a sudden onset of respiratory distress, but are accompanied by a high fever. Croup, an upper respiratory viral infection, typically does not have a sudden onset and often is accompanied by a low-grade fever.

117. B. In the initial steps of assessing and managing the newborn, the most important aspects include clearing the airway of amniotic fluid and making sure that the baby stays warm. The APGAR score should not be relied on as the initial indicator for resuscitation because it is not performed until the child is 1 minute old. Clearly, this is too long to wait before assessment. After the airway has been cleared and the newborn warmed, the respirations, heart rate, and color should be assessed and managed accordingly.

118. C. When the umbilical cord is prolapsed, the infant typically slides down the birth canal and rests on top of the cord, shutting off the infant's own oxygen supply. Placing the mother supine with her hips elevated will cause the baby to slide back into the birth canal slightly, thereby relieving the pressure on the cord.

119. A. Generally, it is safe to clamp and cut the umbilical cord once it has stopped pulsating and the baby is breathing adequately. When the cord stops pulsating, the larger umbilical artery (ductus arteriosis) has constricted, which indicates that the baby is now oxygenating its own blood. If the cord does not stop pulsating and/or the baby is not breathing adequately, the cord should not be clamped and cut and the baby must be kept at the level of the mother's perineum and managed appropriately while en route to the hospital.

120. C. A mass-casualty incident occurs any time the number of injured patients overwhelms your available resources. It is not necessarily defined by the number of patients, but rather your ability to effectively manage them.

121. B. When functioning at the scene of a crime, you must take steps to preserve evidence as much as possible; however, your primary responsibility is to provide appropriate care to the patient. You may need to contact medical control if you need advice, but contact is not necessary prior to initiating the basics of patient care (ie, the ABCs).

122. B. When ventricular fibrillation (V-Fib) is of short duration (ie, witnessed cardiac arrest), immediate defibrillation is the most critical intervention to perform. Prolonged V-Fib (> 4 to 5 minutes), however, results in significant myocardial hypoxia and may be more responsive to defibrillation following a brief (2 minute) period of CPR. 100% oxygen and cardiac drug therapy are important interventions; however, they should not precede defibrillation.

123. A. The most common errors that occur with the AED are the result of operator error, usually because no one made sure that the batteries were fully charged when checking the ambulance at the start of the shift. Because the patient died, you and your partner could be held liable for negligence. Remember, the entire ambulance must be checked by the oncoming shift to ensure that all equipment is functional and that all supplies are present. Even though the preceding crew is morally responsible for not replacing the batteries, the legal ramifications will rest on you and your partner's shoulders.

124. B. Postpartum bleeding is most effectively controlled by massaging the fundus (top) of the uterus. Uterine massage stimulates the pituitary gland to secrete a hormone called oxytocin, which constricts the blood vessels in the uterus and stops the bleeding. Uterine massage should not be withheld until signs of shock are present. The goal is to control the postpartum bleeding in order to prevent shock. Additionally, you should apply supplemental oxygen. Both of these procedures should be accomplished while en route to the hospital. Vaginal bleeding is never treated by placing anything inside the vagina. Careful monitoring of the patient's vital signs should occur and shock treatment initiated if the vital signs begin to deteriorate (ie, tachycardia, cool and clammy skin, hypotension, etc).

125. A. Because a child's head is proportionately larger than the rest of the body, when compared to an adult, the head commonly is the primary site of injury. This is especially true in fall-related injuries, in which gravity causes the head to precede the rest of the body.

126. D. At the peak of the inspiratory phase, the alveoli are filled with fresh oxygen. During the expiratory phase, the oxygen moves from the alveoli to the left side of the heart and the carbon dioxide is exhaled into the atmosphere. The process of oxygen and carbon dioxide exchange in the lungs is called pulmonary (external) respiration.

127. C. Surfactant is a lubricant that lines the alveolar walls. It allows them to expand and recoil freely, thereby allowing for an easy exchange of oxygen and carbon dioxide. Diseases such as emphysema cause destruction in the alveolar walls and a decrease in pulmonary surfactant. This makes the normal process of breathing a struggle for these patients.

128. D. Initial management of a patient with a suspected allergic reaction is to provide 100% oxygen. Positive pressure ventilation may be required if the patient is breathing inadequately. After the airway has been managed, you should inquire whether the patient has a prescribed epinephrine auto-injector. If so, you should contact medical control and obtain permission to assist the patient with the auto-injector.

129. C. Epinephrine possesses dual effects. As a bronchodilator, it relaxes the smooth muscle of the bronchioles and improves the patient's breathing. As a vasoconstrictor, it increases the blood pressure. Diphenhydramine (Benadryl) is an antihistamine that is used to actually stop the allergic reaction.

130. A. If a patient does not have a prescribed epinephrine auto-injector and is experiencing an allergic reaction, which clearly has the potential to deteriorate to anaphylaxis, he or she must be transported immediately, and the airway must be monitored closely while en route. You should consider requesting an ALS rendezvous. The paramedic unit will carry epinephrine on the ambulance and be able to administer it subcutaneously to the patient. Never assist a patient with medication that is not prescribed to him or her specifically.

131. C. Several factors point to a field impression of hypoglycemia (insulin shock). First, the patient is known to have diabetes and second, he took his insulin but did not eat. Because insulin promotes the uptake of glucose into the cells, if the patient does not replace this glucose by eating, the glucose level in the blood will fall to dangerously low levels.

132. C. Insulin is a hormone produced by the beta cells in the Islets of Langerhans of the pancreas. It promotes the uptake of glucose from the bloodstream into the cells where it is used in the production of energy. Glucagon is a hormone produced by the alpha cells in the pancreas. Glucagon stimulates the liver to produce glycogen, a complex form of sugar that is broken down by the body to form the simpler sugar glucose. Glycogen is the body's natural sugar.

133. B. The nature of illness is the medical equivalent to mechanism of injury. Altered mental status should be the suspected nature of illness in any patient with any fluctuation in mental status, which can range from acting bizarre to complete unconsciousness.

134. B. Because ejection from a car is a significant mechanism of injury, after manually stabilizing the patient's head, you should next open the airway using the jaw-thrust maneuver, which involves grasping the angles of the jaw and lifting. You must accomplish this while simultaneously stabilizing the sides of the patient's head with your forearms.

135. C. Although an extrication collar is not the sole means of immobilizing the patient's spine, it must be of the appropriate size in order to prevent flexion/extension of the patient's neck. When immobilizing any patient, whether with a vest-style device or long spine board, the head is immobilized after the torso. Immobilizing the head first will cause potential cervical spine compromise as the torso is immobilized. Determining whether to use a vest-style or a spine board device is based on the patient's condition. Clearly, you must never ask a patient with a potential spinal injury to move the head around.

136. C. You must initially provide manual stabilization by securing the thigh and the tibia-fibula area, which will prevent further injury. Distal circulation should then be assessed. Because of the vascularity of the knee, as well as the presence of major nerves in that area, you should not straighten an injured knee. Joint injuries are immobilized in the position found. If there is no distal pulse, medical control may authorize you to make one attempt to gently manipulate the joint in order to restore a pulse.

137. D. If a wound continues to bleed despite application of a pressure bandage and additional dressings, you must either remove the dressings and apply direct pressure to the site of the bleeding or apply pressure to a proximal pulse point. Packing additional dressings on a severely bleeding wound will only cause the patient to continue to bleed externally into the dressings. If neither of these techniques proves effective in controlling the bleeding, a tourniquet must be used as a last resort.

138. C. Signs of cardiac compromise include pain in the chest or epigastric area, nausea, and an irregular pulse that is either fast or slow. Pain of cardiac origin typically is not reproducible by palpation. Palpable pain to the chest would suggest a musculoskeletal problem, not cardiac compromise.

139. A. Providing appropriate airway support, gathering a SAMPLE history from a family member, and requesting ALS support all would be appropriate measures to take when managing an unconscious patient with a significant cardiac history. The AED is not attached to patients who are not in cardiac arrest; however, the EMT must be prepared to attach the AED.

140. B. The septum is the wall that separates the left and right sides of the heart. There is a septum for both the atria and the ventricles. The carina is the bifurcation point of the trachea, and the mediastinum is the space between the lungs in which the heart, great vessels, and a portion of the esophagus lie. The pericardium is the sac that surrounds the heart and contains serous fluid.

141. B. Prior to assisting a patient with any medication, you must first obtain authorization from medical control. When assisting a patient with prescribed nitroglycerin, you must make sure that the medication is indeed prescribed to the patient and that the systolic blood pressure is at least 100 mm Hg. A detailed physical examination is generally not indicated in a medical patient unless he or she is unresponsive.

142. C. The first step that should be taken after the AED successfully restores a pulse is to assess the airway and continue to provide the appropriate management. After this has occurred, the patient must be transported immediately. Because of the high risk that cardiac arrest can recur following resuscitation, you should not remove the AED. Because the patient now has a pulse, further cardiac rhythm analysis with an AED is contraindicated. Remember that the AED is only used on patients who are pulseless and apneic.

143. C. In contrast with diabetic coma (hyperglycemia), insulin shock (hypoglycemia) has a rapid onset. It is commonly caused when a patient accidentally takes too much prescribed insulin. Insulin is a very fast-acting drug that rapidly causes glucose to exit the bloodstream and enter the cell. Other common causes of hypoglycemia include taking the regular dose of insulin but not eating or taking insulin and exercising heavily.

144. A. In managing a near-drowning patient, you always must consider the possibility of spinal injury. Many water-related accidents occur when a patient dives into shallow water and strikes the head. Water can be aspirated into the lungs but will not cause an obstruction of the airway. Another common finding in near-drowning patients is hypothermia. It is not common for a near-drowning patient to have concomitant internal bleeding unless a traumatic injury occurred prior to the water accident. Spinal injuries are far more common.

145. B. An avulsion is a soft-tissue injury in which a portion of the skin is torn away, leaving a flap of skin. A laceration is a jagged soft-tissue injury that can be caused by glass or other sharp objects. An abrasion is the scraping away of the epidermis, causing oozing of serous fluid from the capillary bed. An abrasion also is referred to as "road rash." An incision is similar to a laceration, but has smooth edges. Scalpel or knives are examples of instruments that would make an incision.

146. C. Hemoptysis (coughing up blood) is a finding that suggests injury to or bleeding within the lungs. Vomiting of bright or dark red blood (hematemesis), suggests gastrointestinal bleeding. Intra-abdominal bleeding would present with signs of shock as well as a rigid, bruised, or distended abdomen. Damage to the myocardium typically does not produce coughing up of blood unless it is associated with lung injury.

147. C. When chest compressions are in progress, the most reliable method of determining their effectiveness is to palpate for a carotid or femoral pulse. If compressions are of adequate depth for the patient's age, you should be able to feel a pulsation during each compression.

148. A. As with most patients, the position of comfort for cardiac patients typically is the semisitting (semi-Fowler) position. You should allow the patient to remain in the position of comfort both during the assessment phase as well as throughout transport.

149. C. Cardiac pacemakers are bundles of nerves that generate electrical impulses and conduct them to the cardiac cells. In the normal, healthy heart, the sinoatrial (SA) node is the primary pacemaker that sets the inherent rate for the heart. The SA node generates electricity at a rate of 60 to 100 electrical discharges per minute, hence the normal adult heart rate of 60 to 100 beats/min.

150. C. The heart has four layers. The inner layer is called the endocardium, the middle layer is composed of muscle and is called the myocardium, and the outer layer of the heart itself is called the epicardium. The pericardium, which is a thin, fibrous membrane, encapsulates the entire heart.

Notes

Notes

Notes

Notes

Notes

Notes

Notes

Notes